Brainstorm

Brainstorm
Copyright © 2025 Susan P. Ryan

All rights reserved under the Pan-American and International Copyright Conventions. This book may not be reproduced in whole or in part, except for brief quotations embodied in critical articles or reviews, in any form or by any means, electronic or mechanical, including photocopying, recording, or by any information storage and retrieval system now known or hereinafter invented, without written permission of the publisher.

Some details such as names and locales have been changed to protect the privacy of individuals. My autobiographical writing emanates from my memory of past occurrences, which may be fuzzy during brainstorm. I have made every effort to be accurate unless providing a bit of satirical comic relief while writing on this serious subject. My purpose is to share hope and encourage fellow travellers on this path toward living a better quality of life.

ISBN Paperback: 978-1-963271-66-9
ISBN Ebook 978-1-963271-67-6

Published by Armin Lear Press, Inc.
215 W Riverside Drive, #4362
Estes Park, CO 80517

Brainstorm

Navigating Life with Chronic Migraine

Susan P. Ryan

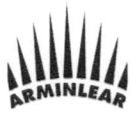

This book is dedicated to the men, women, and children who live in the shadow of chronic pain. May rays of sunshine brighten your days and lift your load.

CONTENTS

Disclaimer		1
Author's Note		3
Foreword by David Sherer, MD		5
Introduction		9
1	Between the Storms—When Life Happens, circa 1965	15
2	The 1970s	19
3	The Migraine Chronicles —Circa Y2K	23
4	Facing Fifty	29
5	The Future is Plastics	37
6	Alternatively	45
7	The Stigma of Migraine	51
8	The Retirement Cure	55
9	The Change of Scenery Cure	61
10	Dr. Lively's Cure	63
11	Pick Your Poison	73
12	Toxic Treatments	77
13	Awakening the Right Brain	85
14	Impatient Inpatient	95
15	In Need of Needling	111
16	The Frankenstein Treatment	117
17	Let's Go Blue	121
18	Monoclonal Antibodies	131
19	The Cannabis Cure	141
20	There Must Be Fifty Ways to Leave Your Migraine	157
21	Tripping on Triptans	171
22	Loving the Buzz	175
23	Balance Your 'Lytes and Dim the Lights	181
24	Pain Is Solitary	185

25	Not Your Mother's Heavy Metal	189
26	Forest Bathing	195
27	Move your Body, Ease Your Mind	199
28	Not So Trigger-Happy	203
29	Eat Right for **Your** Brain	209
30	Why Does Migraine Thrive?	217
31	Change Your Mind	221
32	Reclaim the Brain	227
33	How to Help a Migraineur	233
34	Napping 101	237
35	Smile Awhile	239
36	Twenty-first Century Headache	243
37	Cognitive Impacts	247
38	Patients are Not Generic	251
39	Monoclonal Antibodies 2.0	257
40	Time—Healer or Thief?	261
41	Chronic/Ironic	265
42	Platelets—Perhaps	269
43	TruDOSE™ Redux	275
44	May the Third Time be My Charm	281
45	The Verdict	285
Postscript		293
Glossary of Terms		295
Bibliography		309
Endnotes		313
Acknowledgments		319
Author Bio		321

DISCLAIMER

The information in this book is for general informational purposes and is not intended to diagnose, treat, or cure any disease. Individuals should always consult their health care providers before embracing any suggestions made in this book. Readers' discretion is their sole responsibility.

AUTHOR'S NOTE

Many a trip continues long after movement in time and space has ceased.
—John Steinbeck[1]

These essays represent my journey through migraine, from occasional brainstorm to chronic daily headache. This book is not intended as a replacement for medical advice. I share my experience to provide hard-earned insight with the hope that fellow migraineurs may better advocate for themselves. Though each migraine odyssey is unique, we can learn from one another. Incrementally we can change our minds and our brains, loosen the tethers of pain, and live an improved quality of life. A few names have been changed, but the story is true. It happened to me, and I share so that others may find their path to relief sooner.

FOREWORD

by David Sherer, MD

Migraines are a worldwide problem. According to The Cleveland Clinic, migraine impacts more than 10 percent of the world's population, affecting females three times more than males. It is the third most common disease in the world and strikes 1 in 7 people. To give you a sense of its prevalence as a disease, in the United States alone, 1 in 4 households houses a migraine sufferer.

In her new book *Brainstorm, Navigating Life with Chronic Migraine*, Susan P. Ryan recounts her personal experience with the condition, detailing her pain, treatments, and especially her frustration with this often-disabling malady. In her Author's Note, she lays out her goal in writing the book which, once read, can only help to empower her readers. Her stated aims are "to provide hard-earned insight with the hope that fellow migraineurs may better advocate for themselves."

Many patients who suffer migraine often get shuffled from doctor to doctor, starting with the family physician, then on to the neurologist and finally the pain medicine specialist. Along the way, they receive this or that medication or treatment, attempting to find the right magical potion to alleviate their suffering. Susan's experience was clearly no different.

Rather than writing a dry, clinical tome, she has an engaging and sometimes humorous style, revealing to the reader what was going on in her life and how those events affected her symptoms and her ability to find effective treatments. Indeed, when one examines the lives of many migraineurs (people who suffer migraine), one sees that those affected are often strongly influenced by a number of disparate factors, which may include, the weather, whether the sun is strong that day, work-, financial-, or relationship- related stress, and even odors. Susan reveals how these and other factors impacted her life as a migraine patient, offering insights that non-migraineurs cannot readily understand. In this way, she educates non-sufferers—from both a personal and environmental standpoint—as to what it feels like to be a migraineur. She also relates how a woman's migraine experience can be so different than a man's.

Many migraine patients will readily identify with the author's journey, especially when it comes to treatment. Starting with mere aspirin, and going on to beta blockers, ergotamine, calcium channel blockers, antidepressants like monoamine oxidase inhibitors, triptans, and then botox injections and CGRP (calcitonin gene related peptides) and more, migraine patients over the years have been offered an array of treatments. The author's experience was no different. It can be a daunting task to find the right medication for the person *and the time of life.*

The truly remarkable thing about *Brainstorm* is its breadth. The author is successful in covering just about every angle one

BY DAVID SHERER, MD

can imagine when it comes to migraine, be it symptom description, impact on one's life, treatment options, and even the natural history (or progression) of the disease. I cannot think of another book available that deals with migraine so completely. If you suffer migraine, or know someone does, this book will be an invaluable resource.

—David Sherer, MD
Columnist for *Anesthesiology News*
and author of *What Your Doctor Won't Tell You*

INTRODUCTION

Migraine is the #2 disease-causing disability. Migraine is a primary headache disorder that usually lasts 4–72 hours, accompanied by nausea, vomiting and/or photophobia and phonophobia. The exact cause of migraine is currently unknown.
—World Health Organization[2]

"There is nothing more valuable than your health. That body needs to last for your whole life." I did not appreciate my father's words of caution when I was a young daredevil who climbed trees, played ice hockey, and chased after my older brother and his friends, finding my favorite sport of racing on skis in the ninth grade.

The gravitas in Dad's voice was earned through his participation in a different life. As a young man he served in the U.S. Army, stationed in France and Germany during WWII. Returning home, he survived a near fatal electrocution while working as an electrician at General Motors. Someone in the Livonia

Chevrolet Spring and Bumper Plant snipped off Dad's safety lock which he had taken care to install before climbing a ladder twenty feet to work on high voltage wires. Someone had reconnected the electrical circuit and Dad was jolted out of his shoes and to the concrete floor below, crushing his left ankle. "You will never walk again," said the orthopedic surgeon who attempted to reconstruct his shattered joint in 1957. After spending six weeks in a hospital bed with his left ankle in traction, Dad ignored the surgeon's wheelchair life-sentence and got back to work, though he limped for the rest of his seventy-nine years. Raising eight children, he could not afford to leave work and get by on a reduced income from a permanent disability claim. As a healthy young teen, I was not yet familiar with pain and the absence of good health. I was unable to appreciate Dad's wisdom or his determination to overcome his injury.

Today from my own middle age perspective, I echo Dad's very words about the primacy of health and now realize that time is my second most valued asset. No one who is truly aware has time to waste. Under the cloud of an all-encompassing headache, this migraineur through lowered lids, observes time tiptoeing out the door, not saying goodbye, or planning a return. Living with migraine for almost fifty years, with a background in medicine, I cannot offer a sure cure, though I have taken the bait many times from others who have offered salvation. Each patient is unique and what works for one will not be the universal antidote. Since I have tried most mainstream treatments as well as explored other less travelled tracks, I can offer an insider's guide through this brain-pinched life. I will share parts of my journey in hopes that this insight may help others to find relief from this all-too-common affliction.

The World Health Organization ranks migraine as the #2 disease-causing disability. Yet in 2025, the skull is a still a black box—the inner workings are difficult to interrogate while the patient is alive. The brain is the least understood aspect of humanity. Consciousness, unconsciousness, and the grey area in between are yet to be revealed while crushing pain which emanates from this black box is worthy of moonshot funding. Despite great strides in medicine over the past century, we still lack a cure for headaches and migraine. I believe it is time to focus on understanding the life of migraineurs and improving their quality of life.

Before you start reading, grab a glass of water. Dehydration is the #1 cause of migraine according to neurologists, researchers, and patients. Good quality sleep is probably the next best disrupter of migraine. I recommend that anyone serious about migraine relief should read *Why We Sleep* by neuroscientist Matthew Walker.[3]

I wish you many more pain-free days and nights.

Just a Headache

I wake up feeling fine.
Stretch each arm and leg,
and praise the Lord for His blessings.

Open eyes
  and
    light scalds my retinas,
      reverberates like an aching tooth
        behind red, white, and blue orbs.

        Standing~~~
          the room sways. ~~~
            Seasickness swims~~within.
        Why?
      I have an undeserved hangover
    and I have not done a thing to provoke it.
  Just a headache
which will rip the heart and soul out of my day,
steal words and erase my brain.

It could be worse.
Carry on.

—Susan P. Ryan

chapter 1

Between the Storms— When Life Happens, circa 1965

I'm just glad to be feeling better. I really thought I'd be seeing Elvis soon.
—Bob Dylan[4]

I am twelve years old and reaching for the aspirin bottle in the kitchen cupboard. Dizzy and queasy, I chew two, maybe three tablets, washing the acrid, grittiness down with a glug of milk. I am searching for the quickest absorption of this drug. Chew it up. Gag it down. This is all I have. Nothing matters but pain and erasing it. I squint as the dazzle through dusty windows etches my eyelids with hot acid and I expect to wipe bloody tears from my cheeks. Prior painful experiences were rare, short-lived, painted with mercurochrome, and comforted with band-aids. My parents offered ice tied within a dish towel and pressed it over oozing flesh after a fall off a bicycle, out of a tree fort, or to treat roller skating road rash. But this is different. This is a merciless stabbing through my left eye. It is the dentist's drill without Novocain. The last three doses of aspirin provide no relief, and I know no way to bandage my brain or chill my eyeballs. And now my ears are ringing, tinnitus caused by high blood levels of acetylsalicylic acid (aspirin) and so loud that my world is a buzzing swarm of hornets circling their prey. What are these insects telling me? As I pour out a handful of white vinegary tablets, I consider my options. Do I swallow the entire bottle, or stick with just two more? How much worse can it get? How long will it last? Is this normal? Can I die from a headache? Or maybe that will be my salvation.

Though I am not a depressed adolescent, when overcome with an all-encompassing headache, my thoughts dip toward darkness. My mother is overworked with a houseful of my seven siblings and my headaches are not something to fuss over. "Take an aspirin," I am told each time. Our family is of mostly Irish heritage, and we are expected to be tough since our ancestors lived through the potato famine, endured persecution as Micks, and Catholics to boot. "Give it up for the poor souls in purgatory," I am told whenever I complain. I guess we are born to be martyrs.

Aspirin is the miracle drug in the Ryan household, dispensed for every ailment. Goldfish swimming sideways around their dime store bowl are given a dose. Sometimes they perk up and swim upright and clockwise for a few more days. And if not, they are flushed. With so many children in our home, am I also expendable? Headaches are not considered a real condition by non-sufferers—they are invisible to anyone outside the throbbing skull. Not scarring like chicken pox, splotchy like measles, or jowl-swelling like mumps. They are silent, except for the complaining. And my brain feels damaged. [Note: Aspirin is no longer considered a safe medication for children or adolescents. Though rare, Reye Syndrome can be triggered, resulting in permanent brain damage.]

"It's all in your head," I am told. Indeed. The brain swelling occurs each month while I cycle 'round the moon wearing bulky sanitary pads. As a tomboy, I will not miss out on a thing, lying on the couch clutching a heating pad for cramps like some of my friends each month. Their mothers serve tinned fruit cocktail encased in cool, jiggly Jell-O™ with doses of sympathy. I get some relief for intestinal colic from Paregoric® (camphorated opium) as I ride through the cramps, wearing baggy dark-colored slacks, but brain pain is not ignorable. My gut calms down, but the headache rages on. Opioids do not touch my brain pain, which grabs my attention like nothing else I have encountered in my short, otherwise healthy life.

I recall my Aunt Gertie in her darkened bedroom, admonishing me and my cousins to "please be quiet. Close the door and go take a nap" while she deals with her "sick headache." I connect the dots years later while in pharmacy school. There is a familial tendency toward migraine and two of my father's sisters are fellow sufferers. But it is early. I do not yet have the diagnosis. Migraine has not been attached to my cyclical suffering, and it is not part of my life every single month—yet. In between attacks, I forget all about it.

chapter 2

THE 1970S

Every day may not be good, but there is something good in every day.
—Alice Morse Earle[5]

I will be good for something today.
—Susan P. Ryan

During college, oral contraceptives launch my pinched brain into another orbit. Not only is my monthly cycle predictable, but so is my headache. And it nails me to my bed. The OC hormones are synthetic, high dose, and incompatible with my physiology. They increase the frequency and duration of my migraine. When I complain to University Health physicians who dispense OCs to every coed on the Ann Arbor campus, I am switched from one man-made hormone combination to another without any relief. I begin my own research in the medical school library and decide to take my chances off the pill, with my headaches becoming less frequent, though not vanquished.

My first job after college is detailing drugs for Ayerst Pharmaceuticals, which became Wyeth, and was eventually taken over by Pfizer. Our block-buster drug, Inderal® (Propranolol HCl), the first beta-blocker, was introduced in 1965 to treat cardiac arrhythmias, found helpful for angina, high blood pressure, and is being used off-label in the 1970s for thyrotoxicosis, performance anxiety, essential tremors, anxiety, and migraine prevention. This was the #1 prescription drug for a time and doctors joked about new uses for it. "Can we treat fallen arches and acne yet?" But with widespread use, more information was gathered for other indications. It was a hot drug, much like the current batch of GLP-1 drugs, which were initially approved for Type 2 diabetes. After a few years of use, GLP-1s were found to reduce weight miraculously, help in the management of substance addictions, and possibly improve the outlook for dementia patients. But the side effects of remarkable drugs are minimized or perhaps overshadowed by their marketing potential.

In the late 70s I begin to treat my self-diagnosed migraine, by ingesting twenty milligrams of Inderal twice daily from my sample stash. I soon note a decrease in the severity and frequency of headache, but the side effects become intolerable. My resting heart rate and blood pressure plummet, and I sometimes collapse while getting out of bed. With pharmaceutically slowed circulation, not enough oxygen is reaching my brain, muscles, and organs. Lethargy consumes me for a few weeks until I abandon this experiment. In between headaches, I am vibrantly healthy. Does consuming a drug every day which does not cure and causes dangerously low blood pressure make sense? Lesson learned: some treatments inflict greater morbidity than the original malady. There will be trade-offs in medicine but first do no harm.

In my mid-twenties, newly married, and beginning my career in medical sales, I live pain-free between episodic migraine. If I sleep well, eat on schedule, drink very little or no alcohol, and stay hydrated, I can avoid many migraine attacks. They erupt when I push my limits, skip meals, and especially when I spend time in the sun or become overheated. I am a winter person, preferring layers of clothes to bikinis on the beach. I love winter sports and pray for snow each year on my December birthday. Heat intolerance may be protecting my fair skin from sun damage—an upside to this affliction. And since I am unable to drink more than one alcoholic beverage without causing a headache, I am saved from self-inflicted social and health problems by abstaining. Despite my Irish heritage, I detour from the road so many others have taken in their quest for blissful intoxication, while I trudge soberly in the opposite direction, trying to avoid another brainstorm. I tell myself that the migraine curse may be a blessing.

In a procedure called trepanning, a hole is scraped or drilled into the human skull to treat intracranial maladies including the release of demons. From cave paintings and excavations, it appears that this crude remedy was used during Neolithic times for epilepsy, migraine, and mental disorders. Giving the brain a bit of extra room was the idea. Today trepanation—now called craniotomy—is used to relieve epidural and subdural hematomas and for brain access during neurosurgery. In early times, the bit of bone that was removed during trepanation was worn as a charm to ward off evil spirits. In the throes of a killer migraine, it feels as if my brain is butting up against the confines of my skull. Like a hermit crab, is it my time to search for a replacement container?

chapter 3

The Migraine Chronicles
—Circa Y2K

Those things that hurt instruct.
—Benjamin Franklin[6]

How many times must I learn this lesson?
—Susan P. Ryan

My earliest headache diaries begin around my forty-eighth birthday. Earlier I had been too immersed in my career to keep track of the frequency but now realize that migraine is interfering too often with my life. Having trained in scientific method, I know the importance of measuring the effectiveness, or lack of, for each prescribed treatment. During the month of November, I record seven headache days and take Fioricet®(butalbital), an opioid with acetaminophen, prescribed by my primary care physician.

My current gynecologist suggests that hormone therapy may be beneficial to smooth out fluctuating estrogen levels which may be initiating the headaches.

Here we go again. He prescribes Loestrin® 1.5/30 (progestin and ethinyl estradiol, both synthetic hormones). I hope that the new lower dose OCs will be helpful, not hurtful like the early ones were during college in the 1970s. But holy hell. My headaches increase in intensity and frequency, inflicting misery for three to ten days each month. To stay on the job, I pop the triptan Imitrex®(sumatriptan) and alternate NSAIDs (nonsteroidal anti-inflammatories) Ibuprofen and Naproxen, while pushing through an inky fog of pain and confusion, traveling a four-state territory with long hours in the operating room for my career as a heart valve specialist. I discontinue the OCs and soldier on to the syncopation of my own hormones.

Hot weather melts my brain. I find it difficult to get through a round of golf in Louisville without incurring a migraine in summer months. During August 2002, I record *fifteen headache days*. From my reading of clinical papers, I learn that my headaches are now transformed from "episodic to chronic," probably from overuse of triptans. But how else to get through days with migraine when I need to work? According to the International Headache Society, ". . . chronic migraine is defined as headache occurring on fifteen or more days per month for more than three months." They also state that "chronic migraine affects about one percent of the population and studies estimate that about 2.5 percent of people with episodic migraine will transition to chronic migraine each year." Does this make me feel better knowing that I am not alone in my suffering? Not exactly, but it does make me wonder why more research is not dedicated to this too common debilitating condition since it is the number two reason for disability in the United States.

Neurologists insist that patients maintain a headache journal to quantify the number of days lost to pain and weigh the intensity of pain. Otherwise, insurance companies will not pay for treatments. Some neurologists use a scale of 1-10, others 1-5. I believe most patients under-estimate the frequency of their headaches—I forget the number and quality of headaches I endured last week if I did not record them. But I feel like a hypochondriac writing down every brain attack, listing medications taken, and rating the severity of symptoms. And I find it interesting to note that if I write down the degree of pain while in the throes of migraine, it is always higher than recording it after recovery. Memory of actual pain fades over time. The quantifying and qualifying in a diary are both eye-opening and a disappointment; I have always considered myself a healthy and physically active person and now feel like a malingerer.

The risk factors for chronic migraine as listed by the International Headache Society[7]:

1. *Depression.* The only time I feel depressed is when I cannot escape a brainstorm, and it prevents me from doing what needs doing.

2. *Anxiety.* I am not an anxious person per se, though living in anticipation of the next brainstorm may be nudging me in that direction.

3. *Other pain disorders.* Not yet.

4. *Obesity.* Negative. My BMI is in the 18.5-24.9 range according to the CDC (Center for Disease Control) calculator. (Body mass index = weight in pounds/ height in inches squared x 703).

5. *Asthma.* Only when forced to breathe smoke, though I have seasonal allergies.

6. *Snoring.* I have not heard complaints of my snoring, so I assume I do not snore. However, I have been told that I excel at somniloquy with sales presentations and long-winded nocturnal banter. While rooming with a friend on a bicycle trip, Jean and I both awoke independently to the sound of the other speaking and attempted to engage the other in conversation. One speaker was likely unconscious in REM sleep. Friends in the next room said we chattered all night.

7. *Stressful life events.* Who does not have stressful life events?

8. *Head/neck injuries.* I may have suffered undiagnosed concussions while racing on skis during pre-helmet days.

9. *Caffeine.* My drug of choice.

10. *Acute medication use.* Ding, ding, ding. When you have a headache several days a week and you cannot stay home with an icepack on your noggin in a dark room, it is necessary to obtain relief however you can.

11. *Persistent and frequent nausea.* Only during migraine.

I understand now that the human brain changes from constant onslaught. It is transformed when migraine recurs too often. If a critical quantity of a trigger is detected, the overly sensitive cerebral nerves and blood vessels default to migraine mode. For me triggers seem to be heat, dehydration, barometric pressure change, lack of sleep, stress, bright lights, strong smells—such as in the grocery store detergent aisle, heavy perfume, smoke, loud sounds, dietary—such as raw onions. It may be just one molecule too many which initiates the brain attack. I have not charted moon phases in my headache diary, though hormonal fluctuations are prime suspects for many women. I wonder if I lived beside an ocean instead of Lake Michigan, could I predict high tides? I am frequently asked what causes my migraine. Who knows? That black box may be opened at autopsy, but for now I do my best to live a normal life.

chapter 4

FACING FIFTY

Biology gives you a brain. Life turns it into a mind.
—Jeffrey Eugenides[8]

Indeed.
—Susan P. Ryan

My father died in July 2002. During his five-month hospitalization in Ann Arbor, my mother is engaged in an extramarital affair. With Dad dying and Mom dating, it is a stressful time. I live six hours away in Louisville, trying to help manage my father's care while keeping up with my demanding job. My father experienced a toxic reaction to Celebrex® (celecoxib), an anti-inflammatory prescribed for arthritis. He had watched an advertisement on television for this drug and decided to replace the habit-forming narcotic Darvocet® he consumed each day for many years for his chronic arthritis pain, caused by his on-the-job ankle-smashing accident over forty years earlier. I believe that the United States population was better off before the advent of television ads for prescription drugs. Patients are being marketed to and in turn request promoted drugs from their physicians. If their physician will not prescribe the touted drug, the patient may shop around for another physician. (Darvocet was withdrawn from the U.S. market in 2010.)

After a short time on this new medication, Dad suffers a toxic drug reaction. The prescriber and pharmacist do not reference Dad's sulfa allergy, which should preclude him from ingesting Celebrex, which contains a sulfonamide moiety. His digestive tract from stem to stern sloughs off. The diagnosis is Stevens-Johnson Syndrome. Some patients with this syndrome lose their skin and are confined to burn units. Many lose their eyesight. Dad is in terrible pain, unable to eat, and the SJS reignites as additional drugs cause further reactions. It is so difficult to watch him struggle to live in this awful, uncurable condition. I cannot imagine a worse way to go. With the kind assistance of one of my cardiac surgeon customers, we transfer my dear father from a tiny hospital to the University of Michigan Medical Center. Dad is well-treated but is unable to recover, suffering for five months in the hospital before dying of multi-organ failure at age seventy-nine. Other than arthritis, my father had been healthy before this life-ending drug reaction. I recommend caution and research of any new prescriptions and over-the-counter remedies, making note of allergies and other drugs and supplements one is taking. **Adverse reactions and drug-drug interactions are not uncommon.**

This rough patch may be contributing to my transformation from acute to chronic migraine as I drive back and forth from Louisville to Ann Arbor while covering a sales territory in Indiana, West Virginia, East Tennessee, and Kentucky. For the month of October 2002, I record *seventeen headache days*.

It has been a terrible year for my family, and I decide to do something positive. As I approach a big birthday in early December, I invite my three sisters to join me on a Bicycle Adventures vacation on the Big Island of Hawaii. Using frequent flyer miles, I treat us all to eight days of *ai no kea*—no worries. We leave home on Thanksgiving Day and celebrate my 50th birthday with a week of bicycling in paradise, including the 100-mile Iron Man route. Do I have headaches in this heaven on earth? Yes. While there is no stress, there is sufficient heat on the tropical island to nudge my sensitive brain over its edge. I ride all day, staying hydrated, while dumping water over my head at rest stops to cool off. But headaches rage on four evenings and I am not able to enjoy birthday beverages offered by my sisters and two friends who join the girls' party. I skip the sunset hike at Volcanoes National Park where my sisters later describe hot sneakers melting off their feet as the sun sinks into the Pacific through an otherworldly glow. Migraine interferes with life, though I do my best to power through.

Just before this trip, I visit my first neurologist, referred by my primary care physician, who says that my escalating migraine frequency warrants the care of a specialist. Doc is a short, roundish bear, whose puffy paws attach electrodes to my scalp with a wet adhesive. I flinch while globs of cooling concrete ooze through my freshly coiffed hair and drip down my neck. He says, "You can wash out the cement when you get home. Just relax and close your eyes for thirty minutes." He dims the lights, and I push back in a recliner while the EEG interrogates my brain. It is my lunch hour, and I am dressed for success and considering my afternoon appointments. Sporting punk hair with a business suit and pearls will be interesting in Louisville. I sigh and try to relax in the darkened room, stretching my hands over the torn armrests, resigned to my tethers. "No signs of epilepsy" reports Doc as he scans the EEG strip. Is epilepsy even a consideration without any seizure-like symptoms, or is this a strategy to bill for something that is not measurable? I understand that in both epilepsy and migraine the brain is hypersensitive, though migraine is not known to cause seizures. There may be some crosstalk inside the black box.

I begin Dr. Steiner's migraine treatment, Fioricet, an opioid with acetaminophen, (which my primary care doctor had prescribed earlier) alternating with Imitrex®, the first triptan approved to abort headaches. This newer drug works significantly better at tempering my head pain than opioids. Triptans' mode of action is constriction of cranial blood vessels, but they may also precipitate rebound headaches if used more than two or three days per week. I find it tough to stick to this rule while enduring four or more migraine days some weeks. I undergo a CT scan (Computed Tomography) of the brain, with and without contrast dye. No unusual findings. Two more CT scans check out my nasal sinuses since I suffer from frequent sinusitis. Some abnormalities are uncovered, but nothing repairable without inflicting more problems. Lots of radiation absorbed; are these tests worth the risk?

In January 2003, while visiting my mother in Michigan, her cloud of Giorgio® perfume shoves me off a cliff. The ensuing migraine is unrelenting in its intensity despite my best pharmaceutical efforts along with an icepack, dark room, and focused deep breathing. I call the neurologist for a follow-up visit and a new slew of drugs.

While awaiting the next neurology appointment, I meet with Dr. Odell, OMD (Oriental Medicine Doctor) for acupuncture. He starts me on supplemental magnesium, feverfew, and Vitamin B-2. He advocates a "no gluten, no dairy diet and you must avoid tyramine-containing foods." He has me read "Eat Right for your Blood Type" and I discover that I have been mostly following my recommended Type A diet: agrarian, agricultural.

I continue weekly massage therapy with Julie and add the antinausea drug Phenergan® (promethazine) to the Imitrex. Doc starts me on Depakote ER500mg® (divalproex sodium) at bedtime as a preventative. This is an anticonvulsant and is also used to treat bipolar disorder. A "brain" drug; I think, what the hell? Might as well try it for migraine prophylaxis. May it tame my overreactive brain.

By March 3, I experience my first Raynaud's symptoms—a side effect of Depakote. My fingers and toes flush and blanch red, blue, and white. They are extremely cold—even indoors. This is caused by decreased circulation to the extremities, and if left unchecked could result in gangrene. This is a serious side effect. But when I call Steiner to report my new symptoms, he responds "continue on Depakote and call me back in a month." I suffer *five headache days* in March. Alleluia. But in April, I clock *eighteen days with migraine*, and I am now contending with Raynaud's, something that I endure to this day. I wear gloves most of the time: open fingers for typing, and glove liners under mittens while outdoors in temperatures below fifty degrees. I sleep with an electric heating pad across the foot of my bed, otherwise I cannot fall asleep with icy toes, even with wool socks and down booties. My primary care physician tells me to keep my torso warm, so I begin wearing vests. May, *twelve headache days*, June, *seventeen headache days*. On July 1, Steiner has me wean off Depakote though my side effects continue without the drug. I begin Topamax® (topiramate), another antiseizure medication, as a migraine preventative. This is currently an off-label indication. Initially I am optimistic after reading some early studies of the drug, but in September, I rack up *twenty days with migraine*. As Steiner directs dosage increases, the side effects ramp up: significant weight loss, no appetite, numbness and tingling in hands and feet, diarrhea, slowed thinking, difficulty concentrating, memory impairment, fainting, altered sense of taste. After dropping ten pounds in a short time, friends ask if I have cancer or am I fasting for a modeling career. I have no appetite and forget to eat. My cognitive function is so poor that I cannot remember the names of people I see every week. It is especially daunting to find I am unable to answer technical questions while standing in the operating room and surgeon-customers install my company's heart valves. Sometimes I step away from a patient's open chest and arrested heart to seek advice on the phone from a cardiac surgeon friend. This is not right.

    Whenever I call the neurologist to complain about side effects without reduction in frequency of migraine, he orders me to increase the Topamax dosage and call back in two weeks. He could have used a recording for his rote instructions. Is Doc as frustrated as I am with my failure to respond to treatment, or perhaps, does he not care? I am another nuisance patient. In March 2004, my headaches are averaging over *fifteen days per month*. I am overtaken by migraine for more than 50 percent of my time and the side effects are intolerable on Dopamax. Doc switches me from Imitrex to another triptan, Frova® (frovatriptan), which has a longer half-life. He adds Aleve 500mg® (naproxen sodium) to be taken with the triptan.

In July, I am prescribed a steroid, a Medrol Dosepak® (dexamethasone) to break up a stagnant brainstorm. Doc continues to tinker with the dosage of the abortive meds and tells me to "get some exercise." I shake my head as this 5'5 two-hundred-pound physician, glued to his squeaking office chair, tells me to exercise more. In between migraine eruptions I ride a few times each week with the Louisville Bicycle Club. The rides are 15-100 miles in length through the hilly countryside surrounding the city. I am in great shape except for migraine and the mounting side effects from his so-called treatments.

But I feel that my life is being overtaken by pain, so I begin weekly visits with a therapist to talk about it. Dr. S suggests a medical leave from work to get my headaches under control. My career will be over if I take more than a vacation and I plan to work until age 55 to receive guaranteed medical benefits. Who could afford living in the migraine milieu without insurance? An alternative medical provider starts me on progesterone cream for several days each month, trying to even out the ebb and flow of monthly hormone levels. It is a good strategy, but it does not move the needle.

chapter 5

THE FUTURE IS PLASTICS

Never look back unless you plan to go that way.
—Henry David Thoreau[9]

While out for a drink on a steamy Louisville August eve, my good friend, Missy, RN, introduces me to a cosmetic surgeon, Dr. O'Daniel, at an outdoor bar. Everyone (except me) at the table is sipping chocolate martinis and other high-octane concoctions that will surely ignite my volcano in this heat. While I enjoy San Pellegrino with a lime, Doctor O tells me that he is "not a real surgeon, but a plastic one." I almost miss his joke as I try to function despite my migraine hangover. My brain is not firing on all cylinders. But he catches my attention as he says, "Many of my patients experience remission from migraine following particular facial surgeries." This makes sense. Nerves are damaged during surgery, and with the ensuing numbness, pain may be reduced or eliminated. And the side effect may be a bonus—a more youthful appearance. The only downside is the cost, not covered by insurance even though it is an attempt to stem migraine, and the slight risk from anesthesia. So, in yet another effort to reclaim my life, I undergo blepharoplasty and brow lift at this surgeon's suggestion. Even if the headaches continue their current trajectory, the pain lurking beneath my unwrinkled brow is easier to miss. Doc O does not go for major alterations, but I am asked by friends not-in-the-know if I just returned from vacation after the postsurgical swelling subsides. There is not an obvious change in my appearance, but it is worth a few uncomfortable days. With fingers crossed, I enjoy a reduction in number of headache days.

Pre-op: September, *ten days,* October, *eleven days.*

Post-op: November, *one day,* December, *two days,* January 2005, *two days.* Woo-hoo! A ten-day New Zealand Bicycle Adventures vacation in mid-January may be resetting my numbed brain. With less sensory input from severed facial nerves, my cranial neurons may also be enjoying a wee holiday. I am utterly changed during this trip, away from high adrenaline job stress 24/7. My current needs are breathing, riding, laughing, eating, and sleeping. I enjoy flirtatious attention from a fellow cyclist. Unfortunately, he is another lawyer, and not my first choice after two ex-husband attorneys. Inching toward forty, he says he is looking for the mother of his future children. Apparently, he has not guessed my age. Ha. It is good for my ego to stare down the handsome blue eyes of youth and maturely decline his offer to share tea in his single room.

During this trip I find sleep easy and so refreshing. I share a room with Sayoko, a friend from LA I met on a bicycle trip in

Hawaii. With our group of ten cyclists and three guides, we climb mountains on two wheels in the sweetest air and dazzling landscapes. Each day I am cycling through a movie. Scarce motorized vehicles, verdant rainforests, snowy peaks, and sheep traffic jams give me a chance to savor serenity. It is paradise for this cyclist, and it may be the best medicine yet for me. Can I move here? I find time to reflect on my life, driven and successful, but lacking something. Though the terrain is rugged and the saddle chafes, pedaling in NZ is freeing for me. While acclimating to left side of the road riding, we cover 19 miles the first day while our expert guides tweak our bikes for the journey ahead. The miles mount with 48 the second day, 76 miles, 86 miles, and then a so-called free day.

I am swept along with the crowd to the acclaimed glacier hiking at Franz Josef. Not a fan of heights and against my better judgement, I strap crampons to my boots, wield an ice axe for the first time, and feel anxious as we are roped together. Does this mean we all fall together? All for one? I inch upward trying to keep up with the group. I am last victim on the line, holding up the ascent with my tentativeness. The second to last person begins sliding toward me as one of her crampons fails. It dangles from her foot as she says, "sorry." Gravity drops her into my personal space, her dripping boots beside my running nose. As I try to grip the vertical ice face with my fingernails through thin, silk glove liners, I pray for claws. I am paralyzed. "I want to go down. Now."

A guide unhooks me from the conga line and talks me down from a few stories of height. When I am back on *terra firma*, I decide that this is one hill I do not have to conquer. I do not need to prove to myself or anyone else that I can do this. I do not want to. I can say no. From the ground I hike with another wise cyclist who eschews ice climbing. A guide points out caving, where a refrigerator-size piece splits from the glacier and crashes nearby. I jump. Litigious U.S. attorneys would require ice climbers to sign twenty-page waivers. A public venue for glacier climbing would likely be outlawed in many states. But it is popular here in the birthplace of bungee-jumping. And this option is also offered to our Bicycle Adventures group a few days later.

Learning that I can refrain from participation is a relief. Maybe I will dial back stress-inducing activities in other areas of my life. When I get home, I will reduce unnecessary business trips such as travelling to conventions and sales meetings. Maybe. But I think about retiring from my intense career while I can still enjoy this type of active adventure. I skip the high-speed jet boat ride and bungee jump option due to a blooming migraine and perhaps a newfound strength to say, "no thank you." A soak in sulfurous hot springs after a massage and a liter of NZ glacier water during happy hour are perfect for me. I do not feel too deprived missing out on NZ Sauvignon Blanc.

The next day we ride 71 miles to Lake Moeraki and spend two nights at my favorite place on earth, the Lake Moeraki Wilderness Lodge. Dear Lord, let this be my final destination. Kayaking on the lake and hiking a few miles to the coast, we see floating feathers from penguins, who have recently departed for their summer migration to Antarctica. The wind howls between vertical rocks rammed into the beach, resembling Stonehenge. The roaring breath from the Tasman Sea is too loud for conversation. Speechless, Sayoko and I smile and point and laugh as we absorb negative ions from this joyful place.

Malcolm, the manager at the Wilderness Lodge, takes our group on an 11pm hike along a deserted road to view glow worms hanging out in their worm-fashioned hammocks in shallow caves. The night sky wheels overhead, glittering with Southern Hemisphere constellations. During an undergrad astronomy class at the University of Michigan, I saw these stars only on charts. It is a thrill for me to stand knee-deep in the Tasman Sea, observing these ancient tears in the universe from the other side of the world.

Overnight a storm tattoos the steel roof of the Wilderness Lodge and in my dreams, I float off on a river of rain toward the sea, clutching my mattress, relishing the ride. In the morning Sayoko and I wade through several inches of rain flooding the parking lot and we miss breakfast due to our oversleeping. It was the best rest ever after a day of playful relaxation in paradise. We shake out wet jackets and shoes and clip into pedals on our aluminum steeds for a 97-mile ride. The high point is a tough climb over Haast Pass. On the downhill, riding on the left edge of the road above a deep drop off, I am flying. I say to myself, if my front tire blows, it will be like Thelma and Louise meeting destiny in the canyon below. Sayoko rides beside me and we are both intent on our mission—to stay upright and avoid being swept off the face of the earth. One of the fellows comes from behind and rides beside Sayoko. We are now three abreast on a holy descent. Brian yells, "We're flying 58 miles per hour." My grin feels permanent.

After the next steep climb, I am overflowing with endorphins and hand my bicycle over to the guide to load onto the van. He asks, "Aren't you going to enjoy your well-deserved downhill?"

"No thanks." It was exhilarating to experience that naked speed, balancing my body as one with the bicycle. But I do not need to cheat fate again. I do not need to try for a 60 mph downhill on this slightly steeper descent. As the gal who does not pass up opportunities, I am reforming. I am looking for what is best for me. It is becoming easier to say no.

On February 1, back home in Louisville, I feel well enough to donate blood, something I had stopped doing because of migraine. Life feels better and I feel good enough to optimistically add another active vacation to my schedule. In October 2005, I join nine adventurers on a five-day hike into the Grand Canyon, camping on the Havasupai Reservation. I survive with three migraine-days during the expedition yet feel grateful for the privilege of living outside while inside this wonder of the world for a few days. But my brainstorms wave their ugly flag for eleven days in October. Back to double digits. Rats. The magic of the Southern Hemisphere respite has evaporated. Perhaps it is time to relocate.

With suboptimal cognitive function in this pharmaceutically induced fog that is my current life, my attention deficit disorder kicks into overdrive. In February I am prescribed a "baby dose" of Strattera® (atomoxetine, an adrenergic uptake inhibitor) by my primary care provider to help me concentrate on my job. On the ADD test, I tick enough boxes to qualify for a cursory diagnosis. The neurologist runs another EEG. I suppose this testing is a good moneymaker for a neurology practice, but how is it useful for a migraineur? No pathology found, nor expected, as I enjoy a midday catnap and Medusa-like hairdo, courtesy of the neurologist's mud adhesive. During the shortest month of the year, I record *twenty migraine days*. To abort the onslaught, I ingest yet another round of steroids while worrying about the possible side effect of osteoporosis. I hear my spine crumbling. Doc increases Dopamax, weans me off Frova, substituting Lorcet® (hydrocodone with acetaminophen). The opioid is less effective than placebo. I agree that too frequent use of the triptan is most likely causing rebounds, but what options do I have with a migraine nearly every freakin' day?

One of my friends is going through a divorce and I offer to store anything she might want out of the way until she can move from the marital home. She brings over some jewelry and a handgun which I stow in a back closet. Whenever I have an especially tough week, I joke that it may be time to purchase bullets. I am not suicidal, but I feel at times that I might die from the headaches.

In March, against my reservations from prior experience with this drug, the neurologist adds a beta blocker to the armamentarium. This class of drugs treats cardiac arrhythmias, angina, hypertension, and essential tremors. Since my blood pressure is normally 90/60, the 60mg of Inderal LA® lays me out on the floor. I cannot get a BP reading on my sphygmomanometer. It is déjà vu all over again, as Yogi Berra said.

I call my primary care physician and receive a referral to a headache clinic in Chicago. No matter where one lives, all experts are located out of town. Since I have exhausted all the tricks of the Louisville neurologist, it is time for a new migraine manager. Dr. N, a neurologist who specializes in headaches, does not require an EEG but sends me in a taxi for a STAT MRI with contrast dye which shows no pathology. I almost hoped he would locate an abnormality, something to pin the blame on, something to extract, and cure me. He prescribes Norflex® (Orphenadrine) 100mg, a muscle relaxer at bedtime, Pamelor® (nortriptyline, a tricyclic antidepressant), and MigreLief®, a supplement containing Magnesium, Riboflavin, and Feverfew. Along with the triptan Frova, I have prescription-strength nonsteroidal anti-inflammatory Ponstel® (mefenamic acid) as abortive treatments.

The following month I experience *no headache days*. Is this a placebo effect from this magical clinic or a cure? The next month May, *two headache days*, June, *six days*. But by August I am again nudging the chronic mark with *twelve headache days* and hover in this range for the rest of the calendar year. In December I have three impacted wisdom teeth removed. Many alternative medical practitioners recommend this for migraine relief, and I am disappointed to find that it makes no difference for me. I have not experienced any issue with these hidden teeth but recall my mother undergoing this procedure at age seventy-nine to prevent erosion of her mandible. I am not well-versed on dental procedures but figure it is worth a try at age fifty.

When I fly back to Chicago for a return visit to the clinic in early January, the neurologist listens to my complaints about side effects and increasing days of wrestling with the monster. He gives me an intramuscular injection of Toradol® (ketorolac), an NSAID, (nonsteroidal anti-inflammatory drug) to take the edge off my migraine in progress and writes a prescription so I can jab myself at home. Frequent use of oral NSAIDs is tearing up my gut; I have developed a gastric ulcer, not uncommon for chronic pain sufferers. IM injections bypass the gut and are better tolerated, though the injections are painful and inconvenient for self-administration in the gluteus maximus. I live with Hamlet, a sweet, black cocker spaniel, who has not mastered enough dexterity to help me out.

chapter 6

Alternatively

The natural healing force within each of us is the greatest force in getting well.
—Hippocrates[10]

On January 15, 2006, I meet Dr. B, a Complementary Medicine MD who embraces both Eastern and Western medicine. Doc asks me to walk down a long hallway ahead of him as he monitors my gait. I am self-conscious and wonder what he suspects. A brain tumor? Doc spends two hours talking and listening to me, so unlike others in the medical establishment. He asks about my IBS-queasy gut that I have had forever, beginning with a colicky first year according to my parents. Doc says a "leaky gut" is preventing absorption of minerals, specifically magnesium. He suggests that I may be allergic to dairy and wheat and asks me to refrain from these foods for six weeks. I drop fifteen pounds and look like a poster child for an anorexia clinic except for the muscular legs of a long-distance cyclist. Doc prescribes Permeability Factors®, a liquid supplement of trace minerals, along with Bach Rescue Remedy®, a homeopathic mainstay.

Doc runs a slew of labs and announces that my hormones are in the menopausal range, as expected at my age, and finds that my total cholesterol is higher than the desirable 200 or less at 236. So, not so good. Fortunately, my CRP level is low, a good thing since C-reactive protein (produced in the liver) levels rise in response to inflammation. Halleluiah for a single piece of good news. Doc implants Sotte Pelle® pellets with a gun-type device. I think he is more nervous that I am as he shoots this bioidentical hormone replacement underneath the skin on my right flank.

Doc hands me different supplements and herbs, one at a time, and presses down on my outstretched arm to determine which may be the most effective treatment based upon my muscle strength while holding the ingredient. This woo-woo technique is a first for me. It was never discussed in pharmacy school. He prescribes Butterbur and some Chinese herbs that give me a rash. When I show up in his office late on a Friday afternoon without an appointment, caught in the teeth of a raging migraine after a chiropractic visit, Doc offers me a bolus of 50mg magnesium IV. The infusion causes immediate hot flushing, dizziness, and a melting of pain. Relief is short-lived. It lasts until I arrive home, five miles away. But I take his relaxing recommendation of an Epsom Salts bath before bedtime each night. Absorbing magnesium sulfate through the skin is soothing. I am increasing magnesium in my body without bowel upset and I sleep more soundly.

The next month I fly to Washington State for six days of

cross-country skiing, starving on the restrictive diet with an amped metabolism. While the rest of my fellow skiers devour hefty carb-loaded sandwiches on the trail, I nibble lettuce wraps and wonder how I will muster the energy to ski uphill to the lodge ten miles away. I am running on fumes. At dinner, my new friends scarf my share of the breadbasket, as well as waffles each morning. I am food-envious but try to stay on the diet. My mother says I will look svelte in my coffin. *Ten headache days* in February.

In March, I get up in the middle of one night and pass out, hitting my hip on the edge of my sleigh bed while saving my head from further damage. I recount my diet of the prior day and decide that I may have ingested too much sugar. It was an unconscious celebration of forbidden foods at the conclusion of the punitive diet. My dinner was popcorn, ice cream, Greek yogurt, peaches, and homemade granola. Not a normal menu for me and a lesson learned: blood sugar matters. I now try my best to keep it as steady as possible, since spikes and resultant drops are migraine triggers and may cause me to faint.

In April Dr. B draws labs again to assess hormone levels. He prescribes progesterone 200mg at bedtime. I undergo ALCAT® allergy testing, searching for food sensitivities. My Food Sensitivity Test warns of my "severe intolerance to cashew, peanut, thyme, and trout." I am deemed "moderately intolerant of apple, cane sugar, cauliflower, cayenne pepper, date, egg yolk, eggplant, flaxseed, fructose, garlic, honey, lamb, millet, navy bean, oat, oyster, pineapple, psyllium, salmon, shrimp, squash, tapioca, tomato, turkey, walnut, white potato. I am told to limit brewer's yeast, mushroom, barley, malt, wheat, cow's milk, banana, black eyed peas, cabbage, carrot, chickpea, corn, crab, fig, goat milk, halibut, lettuce, mustard, olive, onion, pear, rye, sardine, snapper, sole, tuna." The list makes me hungry, and I wonder how I can avoid these foods while traveling for business every week.

In May, I head back to the Chicago clinic with a blood pressure of 90/60, tingling and numbness in fingers, and photosensitivity. *Ten headache days* that month.

I am raising money for charity and looking forward to riding in the MS 150, a 150-mile bicycle ride to be held June 2 and 3 in central Kentucky. With the weather forecast for temperatures in the mid-nineties, I am concerned about surviving the ride with my heat intolerance. On the second day, I arrive at the last rest stop to refill liquids and I pass out in the shade of an oak, unable to ride the last seven miles. Even though my friends empty their water bottles on my hot head and order me to get back on my bike, I cannot crawl over the finish line. The migraine wins this time, 143 miles into the ride.

Doc B prescribes a new supplement, L-Theanine, a green tea extract, touted to promote relaxation without drowsiness, along with probiotics daily and digestive enzymes with each meal. He says, "stay on the rotation-elimination diet for three months to heal your gut and reduce headaches." But it is not so easy when you are on the road three or four nights each week for your job, entertaining customers over meals, and sleeping in hotels. July, *ten days*, August, *nine days*, September, *thirteen headache days*.

On October 2, I fly to New Mexico for a girls' weekend of hot air ballooning and art gallery gazing. I am the designated driver while my friends imbibe at lunch and dinner. I manage to keep the car on the road to Santa Fe with "just a headache." I function well on autopilot, thanks to training from my occupational long-distance driving while I note that an elevation-induced headache is identical to a hangover. Without consuming a single Margarita, I am hungover on Sandia Peak.

On October 12, I head back to Chicago for medication adjustments by the out-of-town experts. "Let's decrease Inderal to 50mg/day." Easy for Doc to say while my resting heart rate is 48 beats per minute, and I feel wiped out. I need caffeine to overcome inertia and lots of exercise endorphins to function. We discuss the difference between optimal levels of hormones for me vs. so-called normal levels, as listed by labs and based on studies of 20-30-year-old patients, rather than perimenopausal women. November, *five headache days*, December, *eight days*.

chapter 7

THE STIGMA OF MIGRAINE

Be not simply good—be good for something.
—Mahatma Gandhi[11]

Despite outward appearances, I am trying with every ounce of my being.
—Susan P. Ryan

After twenty-four years of working for Medtronic, Inc., the largest manufacturer of implantable medical devices, and whose motto is "Toward Man's Full Life," I expect the HR department to be a little more empathetic to one of their employees who has been selling millions of dollars of heart valves each year. How many other jobs am I supporting at this company? Whenever my sales territory brings in over $5 million in a year, some of my favorite accounts are reassigned to newer employees. My current boss is not a fan of female employees. He tries to squeeze out women whenever he has the opportunity and refuses to promote a well-qualified technical service rep who I have been mentoring for a few years. From my perspective, territories are unfairly realigned, with the meaty parts going to men. And this manager chooses only male replacements whenever he encourages a woman to leave the company. I am shocked one weekday afternoon when I am instructed to join a conference call with this manager and a human resources representative. The issue is my migraine. I am meeting my assigned sales goals, my customers are fully serviced, and whenever I cannot personally attend a surgical procedure, I schedule a technical rep to cover for me, though I mostly work through my brainstorms. However, I decline to attend a few out-of-town conventions, and a sales meeting or two, but my contribution to the bottom line is not compromised. So, I am surprised when the HR person suggests that I "go on disability until the migraines are over." How wonderful if a cure will occur with a few weeks off work. I consult with an employment attorney and explain my situation. I have planned to work until age 55, to be eligible for full retirement benefits including guaranteed health care. I care about my customers, I do not want to abandon them, and I want to train my replacement. So, I devise a plan. With twelve weeks of accumulated vacation, I offer to work three weeks on, one week off each month until the end of the next year when I will be 55. During the monthly vacation week, I will be on call in case the new rep needs help. When the company refuses my plan, I give twelve months' notice that I will be retiring. The company pays me a lump sum (with tax consequences) to replace the accrued vacation time when what I want is a reasonable transition for my customers and me. The misogynistic boss hires a male rep instead of the very qualified woman I have been mentoring, who knows my customers and product line very well. It is bittersweet to leave, but a relief too.

Those who have not experienced migraine often brush it off with, "I get headaches when I drink too much, too." The migraineurs I know do not choose to over-imbibe if it may incite a hellacious headache, which may last for two to three days. We have no control over the onset of our brainstorms and are often blind-sided when we are working so hard that we do not notice storm clouds congregating over our heads. We look normal, hide our pain most of the time, and tough it out when we would be better served by lying down in a dark room with an icepack and sipping from a thermos of electrolyte solution. Migraine is not "just a headache." And we try to believe that it is, because we have been conditioned by society to believe this.

chapter 8

THE RETIREMENT CURE

The trouble with retirement is that you never get a day off.
—Abe Lemons[12]

Just wish the brainstorm would retire too.
—Susan P. Ryan

January 2008, only *3 headache days*. Yay! Let us celebrate incremental improvement.

It is one month after my 55th birthday and I retire from Medtronic after a twenty-five year-career as a Heart Valve Specialist. This may be the medicine I need, stress reduction. February, *nine headache days*. March, *fifteen headache days*. WTF? *Beware the Ides of March*. Dr. B prescribes Estradiol patches along with Progesterone 100mg to balance my hormones. April, *twelve headache days.* Neurologist N replaces Inderal with Bystolic® (nebivolol), saying, "You may experience fewer side effects since Bystolic is a Beta-1 specific blocker. I look up possible side effects and note *headache,* dizziness, tiredness, fatigue, slow heartbeat, nausea, stomach pain, diarrhea, insomnia, numbness, or cold feeling in hands and feet. I experience these symptoms before taking this drug, but I do not yet have the rest of the list: shortness of breath, rash, fluid retention in the legs. This drug is classified as an antihypertensive, though I have hypotension. I understand that physicians do not currently have many migraine-specific drug choices, but this is yet another questionable option. May, *sixteen headache days.*

A highly recommended chiropractor orders a boatload of expensive X-rays which are taken in his office. It is a red flag for me when a practitioner double-dips. Oh-so-subtly, he manipulates my neck by tapping with a plastic "actuator," which looks like something from a child's doctor kit. It feels mildly annoying and a waste of my time. I feel no benefit from this faux treatment. His subtlety disappears when he next hangs ten pounds of traction from my head to stretch my neck as I lay uncomfortably on a table for ten minutes. This "treatment" elicits a major migraine, and I vomit in the parking lot on the way to my car. I consider crossing him off my list, but in desperation, I give him a bit more time to cure my pain. I visit his office eight times in June and July and received a bill for $2,135. He says that he does not accept my insurance even though I am well-covered by Blue Cross/Blue Shield. I have never been slammed with such an exorbitant bill for so little care. Perhaps BC/BS does not participate with this fellow for good reason. Does this chiro-quacker think the pain of his bill might supplant the pain in my head? I tell pseudo-doc that I will pay what I consider fair, and if he pursues it further, he will be getting a review from me in the *Louisville Courier Journal*. (This is before the advent of YELP and other online raters.) I have met charlatans in many professions and feel it is an apt label for this fellow who attracts crowds of suffering people to his waiting room five days a week. They expect relief, hoping and returning, while he schedules more appointments and empties their wallets. He is a first-class con. I do not know if anyone has been cured in his office, but the crowd continues to limp from the parking lot to this quasi-medical mecca. June, *ten headache days.*

Another sinus infection crops up, stemming from allergy to June blooms. My treatment includes a Z-PAK® (azithromycin) and overcoming a learning curve with a neti-pot. My primary care physician advises me to use sterile saline to flush the sinuses twice each day. I add ¼ teaspoonful of sea salt to one cup of boiling water, allow it to cool to ambient temperature, and concentrate on mouth-breathing while pouring the warm liquid from the neti pot through one nostril and watching it drip out the other, my head tilted sideways. Once I get the hang of it, the water-boarding comparison fades. It is like learning to swim the Australian crawl over a bathroom sink. Do not inhale through one's nose. It is worth the effort since it relieves the facial pressure for a while. In July I begin a fourth antibiotic this year for sinusitis, which surely influences the frequency and severity of migraine since the cranial nerves are so closely associated with the congested and inflamed nasal cavities.

On July 31 I meet Dr. Blevins, ENT, handing him CAT films of my troubled sinuses while describing my lethargy, maxillary sinus pressure, difficulty in breathing while lying in bed, nasal stuffiness, not feeling refreshed in the morning, and requiring afternoon naps. I lack energy for my usual activities and the four rounds of antibiotics wreak havoc on my gut. Blevins sends me to Dr. Jack Wilson, DMD who hands me off to Dr. Creech, an endodontist for a root canal on #3 upper second molar on 8/4. He prescribes Ponstel® (mefenamic acid), an NSAID, and Vicodin ES® (hydrocodone and acetaminophen), an opioid, for tooth-throbbing, plus a round of Penicillin VK® along with ibuprofen 600mg three times daily for a week. I also take the triptan Frova as needed for migraine. If I take the triptan early, it sometimes intercepts the migraine, but since it is only allowed two or three times per week, I tend to reserve it, hoping it is "just a minor headache" until it is too late to silence the pain and quell the overall flu-like feeling.

On August 15, Dr. B administers a testosterone injection, planning to beat my hormones into some type of manly submission. One short-lived benefit: I find that my golf shots are longer off the tee after this performance-enhancing dose. On August 16, I return to the clinic where I am prescribed Zonegran® (zonisamide), a sulfa class drug with anticonvulsant effects. Since I already enjoy the listed side effects of drowsiness, dizziness, *headache*, tired feeling, loss of appetite, weight loss, loss of balance or coordination, I wonder, will these effects be enhanced with this new drug? Do I really need this? At last, I taper off Dopamax and trade out Zanaflex® (tizanadine) for Norflex® (orphenadrine), both muscle relaxers. I record *15 headache days* in August.

Dr. N brandishes his prescription pad and orders dexamethasone to break the rebounding headache pattern. After two doses I feel like Wonder Woman with loads of energy from the steroid burst. Instead of driving home to Louisville from Chicago, I snake my sedan around the south shore of Lake Michigan and begin perusing real estate. I land at a Holiday Inn Express® in South Haven, Michigan. Unable to sleep from the steroids, I pull up Zillow® and Realtor.com® on my laptop and peruse small vacation cottages near Big Blue. In hindsight, I am pretty sure it is the drugs that make me impulsively purchase a 3000+ square foot 1940s colonial one house away from the Great Lake. The location is lovely although the home requires *beaucoup* TLC and updating. My move from my old Kentucky home back to Michigan during the recession of 2008, and newly retired at 55 due to chronic migraine, is precipitated by a root canal which give me a rebounding headache from round-the-clock NSAIDs. This constant head pain, nausea, and dizziness, treated with a mega steroid burst, masks my symptoms, keeps me awake, and imbues me with super-powers, causing me to open my wallet and my heart. I have lived twenty-two years in Louisville, longer than I have lived anywhere else. It is home, but I miss the Great Lakes, my family, and cooler summers. Maybe the move to Michigan will be good for my head too. It is September 2008, and I own two large homes during the great recession; *nine headache days in September*.

chapter 9

THE CHANGE OF SCENERY CURE

A happy life consists not in the absence, but in the mastery of hardships.
—Helen Keller[13]

I consider my life to be more than 50 percent happy. Let's hear it for adversity.
—Susan P. Ryan

My headaches remain in a holding pattern despite the new climate in Michigan: October, *nine days*; November, *ten days*; December, *ten days*; January 2009, *eleven days*; February, *two days*. Bliss. Near perfection for me. March, *six migraine days*. April, *one blessed migraine day*. May, *nine migraine days*. Rats.

Raynaud's Syndrome is formally diagnosed by internist Dr. D in South Haven. My intensely cold fingers and toes persist despite warmer spring weather. June, *one blessed migraine day*. On July 16, I visit Dr. N at the headache clinic in Chicago. He instructs me to taper off the beta-blocker since the headaches are at a "manageable level" and the side effect of low blood pressure causing postural hypotension is the greater of these evils. I may fall from the dizziness it induces. Allergies causing sinusitis, interfere again with my sleep. I swim just before sunset in Big Blue on warm days and acquire a kayak for bird watching and exploring along the Black River. I search for Great Lake shipwrecks below my blue paddling perch.

July, *two headache days*; August, *six headache days*; September, *ten headache days*; October, *six headache days*. November finds me tapering off the estrogen patch and rejoicing without the beta-blocker-induced dizziness. My old Kentucky home finally sells, closing in December after one year on the depressed housing market. Another sinus infection, so a new allergist begins my third round of allergy shots since childhood. December, *ten headache days*; January 2010, *ten headache days*. This is not what I looked forward to while dreaming of retirement. I am not satisfied with this frequency of headache days, this sometimes-lousy quality of life. I am a fixer, not a quitter so I keep searching for my cure. I drive east across lower Michigan to meet my latest healer.

chapter 10

DR. LIVELY'S CURE

Do you love life? Then do not squander time, for that is the stuff life is made of.
—Benjamin Franklin[14]

On the floor behind a mahogany desk, a trio of Marilyn Monroe lithographs leans against the wall beside diplomas in black frames—University of Michigan Medical School, a residency in OB-GYN, professor at Wayne State University, and stacks of others I do not paw through. From the dates of his accomplishments, I peg Doc at about sixty years old. His penthouse office is freshly painted a calming taupe and overlooks a Jaguar dealership several stories below. From an adjacent room I hear Dr. Lively speaking into a phone about an upcoming medical exposé on ABC News.

"They'll call me a crank, a heretic, but I've cured diabetes in men by adjusting testosterone and other hormone levels. *A beat.* Yes, and I've found through my work since 1985, that these treatments are safe and effective, yet the FDA and big Pharma want to shut me down because there's nothing to patent." He pounds on his desk for emphasis. And I jump. A couple waits in an adjacent room. I can hear their murmuring, but not clearly enough to make out their conversation. The phone rings often and Judy, the office manager, pokes her head into the doorway between calls.

"Ms. Ryan, I am sorry for your wait. There is one patient ahead of you. Would you like a glass of water?"

"Sure, thanks," I say while thinking, waiting is not a problem. It gives me time to bolt, and I seriously consider this idea. Though Judy and Dr. Lively appear to be the only employees of the Why Not Wellness Clinic, I am surprised to hear Dr. Lively answer phone calls whenever his administrative assistant is tied up on other lines. During my thirty years in medical sales, I have never observed a single specialist answering an incoming call on an office phone. This duty is never listed in their job description.

After a ninety-minute wait, Dr. Lively strides into his office. He shakes my hand, peers into my eyes, and asks, "How did you hear about me?" His voice rings loud and as clear as a radio announcer's. He is a broad man, with meaty fists that caught lots of babies in a prior medical practice, and his presence fills up the room. He oozes something I cannot yet pinpoint. Confidence?

"I read your textbook and wondered if you might be able to help me," I say while noting that his red bow tie matches his sneakers and complements his polka dotted socks that peek out beneath his tailored slacks when he crosses his legs. "I've tried most traditional and alternative types of migraine treatments without relief, just loads of side effects."

While scribbling notes, he continues to nod as I relate attempts by prior physicians using mainstream methods to reduce the frequency and severity of my migraine attacks. After taking my medical history, Doc escorts me into a treatment room, where he multitasks as scribe, nurse, and medical technician. He props my arm upon a folded bed pillow, snaps on a tourniquet with one hand, thumps on my left median cubital vein, and then, expertly withdraws five vials of blood. He labels them and fills out relevant paperwork.

"What kind of insurance do you have, Ms. Ryan?"

"Blue Cross Blue Shield of Minnesota."

"Well, your good news is the blood work might be covered. The bad news—the rest of today's fees will not. But it's not all bad, because *I will cure you of migraine*. You haven't scared me a bit with your medical history." No one has yet uttered such a bold pronouncement to me. I really want to believe him, but a large grain of salt lodges in my throat, and I cough.

"Why do you say Blue Cross will not pay these claims?"

"It's a long story, but I'll give you the highlights." Doc leans back in his Aeron™ chair and looks beyond me. For a few minutes, he seems to be transported from the treatment room. My eyes fix on his red sneakers, and I wonder in the silence between us if this may be my moment to exit too. He speaks at last. "My first wife filed a fraud claim against me through Blue Cross, and now this corporation seems to hold something personal against me. They won't accept claims from my office. She's nothing but an anorexic sociopath who enjoys tormenting people." As he says this, he unsheathes two ginormous syringes, attaches extremely long needles, and loads them with three different drugs for me: a steroid, an analgesic, and lidocaine (a numbing agent). I try to ignore the waving needles as he readies the concoction. I flash back to a procedure in an animal lab, where I assisted cardiac surgeons by holding the hooves of a large mammal which never regained consciousness. I think it was a female goat in Dayton, Ohio.

It is a grey February day in Michigan with temps in the teens and I have dressed for the climate rather than the event, in lots of layers. "Do you want me to take off my turtleneck?" I ask.

"That's a great idea. You want a gown?"

"Yes, please."

He rummages through a cabinet and comes up empty handed, while I shiver on an icy stool in my Maidenform™ bra.

"You know I'm a gynecologist—so don't be too modest." And a nurse, and a Jack-of-all-trades.

"Can you lift your hair?"

My muscles guard against his assault. Goosebumps erupt along the chilling splash of alcohol from mid-spine up to my hairline. Unnerved by the antiseptic aroma, I flinch when the first needle pierces the flesh just beneath the skull to the right of my spine. Pain sears through my core and bounces to and from my brain as he squirts the initially gelid then suddenly very warm block into a tight knot of muscle. Heat boils the trigger point of nerves, and I clench my teeth, willing this fire to unlock my pain. He directs his aim down along the right side of my thoracic spine, repeating more deep jabs, instructing me to lift my arms to position the muscles for further stabs and then "shoulder blades together for the last injection on the right side." These are his last words before my world collapses into a dark, buzzing tunnel.

"Dr. Lively, I'm going down," I mumble as gravity draws me toward a face plant on the terrazzo floor. He withdraws the needle and catches me with my nose below my knees. When the buzzing fades and the black veil lifts from my eyes, I focus on his red shoes just inches away. He assists me to the exam table where I recover for a few minutes, with cool compresses draped over my face and neck. I sip tepid water from a paper cup and try to psych myself for the left-sided injections yet to come. I might be lopsided if I flee now with only half of the treatment on board. He leaves the room, and I hear clattering down the hall. In a while, Lively returns.

"Let's have lunch before continuing. I have some Chinese leftovers from my dinner last night. Meet me in the kitchen."

I toss on my jacket and wobble after him in a daze. Grateful for the impromptu meal, I wolf a plateful of microwaved stir-fried beef with peapods over sticky brown rice while sitting at a card table with my latest healer. Over lunch, Doc launches into a diatribe: "The Director of the FDA personally called to shut down one of my clinical trials. He threatened to revoke my medical license if I persisted. I should've been scared, but instead I switched from a randomized trial to a stepped one, where my protocol was used only when patients failed to get relief from migraine after five standard treatments. My protocol was number six. Later, one of the discussants at a medical conference asked me why I didn't do a randomized trial. Duh! How can medicine advance when our hands are tied by a bunch of lawyers?"

I am surprised to hear him confiding in me, a new patient. Is it because of my medical background, or does he share equally with other patients? Though he is relating an interesting story, I want to discuss my prognosis. I am the patient here and footing the not insignificant bill that my insurance will not cover.

"Dr. Lively, how sure are you that stopping my current treatments and beginning your regimen will decrease my headache frequency?"

"You will be cured," he says for a second time and resumes bashing lawyers, the medical establishment, the FDA and ex-wives. After lunch, he tosses paper plates, washes forks, and scrubs his hands for the rest of my procedure. He is doctor, nurse, med tech, scribe, chef, and busboy. I am surprised to see this well-trained physician rinsing silverware. The surreal scene makes me wonder. Am I still unconscious?

"No charge for lunch today," he says.

"My treat next visit."

Back in the exam room I resume a vulnerable position. Fueled by bad Chinese food, and desperate for a less painful existence, I feel fortified for the second assault. I try to believe that this physician is the answer to my prayers, much like I believed in many others before him. There was the Louisville acupuncturist who inserted thin needles all over my body, searching for healing pathways. After several months of soothing Eastern flute and lute music and kindly care without relief, I moved on. My chi would not focus. Was it my overriding ADD? I tried three more acupuncturists without success, interspersed between visits to traditional Western medicine physicians. I endured rounds of chiropractic manipulations: four practitioners in total. Their methods seemed to inflict more damage than alleviation and I often left their offices feeling worse than before the appointment.

Massage therapy gives me relief for up to 48 hours; oh-so-short, but sweet. So, unless I acquire a live-in masseuse with very good hands, it will be difficult to ascertain if every other day massage may be my winning ticket. I once spent five days at a clinic in Florida with a famous massage therapist, Paul St. John. I was referred by my dear friend and massage therapist Julie Harper to this founder of Neurosomatic Therapy. The treatment was soothing and focused on my noggin, but the effects were transitory. Perhaps I needed a longer stay at the spa, but my career was at its apex and a week was the maximal time I could put my life on hold. I remember a piece of Paul's advice which I still revere. He said, "Susan as a Type A+, you need to find a way to dial it down a notch. Instead of perfection, strive for excellence." I am still working on this. Today, I embrace massage therapy as a palliative, not curative migraine treatment. I currently schedule a ninety-minute therapeutic massage every other week, focusing on migraine and degenerative spine issues. Based on my many experiences with massage, I suggest that fellow migraineurs find a well-trained and skilled therapist for regular sessions. There are no side effects.

During the second half of the treatment, I remain conscious, but edgy. The left side is not less painful or frightening, but it is difficult to pass out again so soon, especially after ingesting the sodium and MSG-laden (monosodium glutamate) meal. My blood pressure may be slightly elevated by Doc's prescribed lunch. My mind wanders between shocking jabs, and I wish that my mortal self could follow. An out-of-body experience may be just the thing to escape this torture. Perhaps my healer is going to scare the migraine out of me with his menacing needles. It does seem a bit like an exorcism. I survive the left-sided attack, feeling limp as I pull on my turtleneck sweater. A nap under a down comforter is what I crave. I calculate the distance to my cozy bed.

"Dr. Lively, will I be okay to drive? It's about 200 miles to my home this afternoon."

"Sure, just sit for a bit and let the medicine take effect."

I wait a few minutes for my miracle cure, then, I float to the appointment desk.

"I'm glad you've eaten lunch, so you won't pass out again when you see the bill. It's expensive, but it will be worth it," Judy says. She totals the charges on a calculator and schedules my return visit in three weeks. The bill is over $1,200 for the initial office consultation, nerve blocks, and trigger point injections. Thank goodness for Blue Cross which covers the blood work. I sail outside into a fuzzy world with a handful of prescriptions, instructions, and renewed hope for a headache-free life. ***Will I be cured?*** For a three-hour office visit including lunch, the tab is comparable to that of many lawyers who had exploited me without a shred of compassion, and certainly they never shared their lunch. Sharks never share.

I buckle into my car seat, shift into drive, and run over the curb in front of me. Not a good move on the second floor of a parking garage. Driving home may be a challenge. I run over another curb on the way to the attendant's booth. Time out. I drive through a nearby Starbucks for a double-shot decaf latte. I am under doctor's orders to reduce caffeine, especially after 3pm.

I feel . . . strange. My neck and shoulders move without

their usual stiffness and an adrenalin-like buzz propels me. I set the cruise control once I escape city traffic and stay in the middle lane, praying for a safe trip. On the drive, I stop and make a few attempts to fill the latest prescriptions. No luck. Three pharmacies are out of stock for my new medications, best characterized as snake oil, placebo, and hemlock. I arrive home fourteen hours after my morning departure. I rub the dull throb on the right side of my neck and wonder if I look any different. Bruises are blooming in the mirror as I change into pajamas. Am I healed? Is this my cure? Only time will tell if Dr. Lively is a genius.

Nothing changed for me, so at my return visit, I accept a handful of syringes containing testosterone for self-injection and Danocrine® (danazol), an androgen, to suppress ovarian function. I am relieved that I do not grow a beard and thrilled to see my golf drives are yards longer. Doc increases my current regimen of Vitamin D-3, Neurontin® (gabapentin), an anticonvulsant also used for nerve pain, and adds Aldactone® (spironolactone), a diuretic, that may also help to balance hormones, plus Armour Thyroid®, even though my thyroid blood levels are in the normal range. Doc directs me to a compounding pharmacy for an anti-inflammatory/muscle relaxant cream of ketoprofen 20 percent and cyclobenzaprine 2 percent to be applied to the forehead. Everything is off label and a stab in the dark. Perhaps one drug from column A, one drug from column B. Will the side effects be as random?

February, *eleven headache days*; March, *nine headache days*; April, *five headache days*; May, *eleven headache days*, June, *nine headache days*; July, *twelve headache days*; August, *fifteen headache days*. Not even a hint of a cure, though negligible side effects. I try to count every blessing.

In another quest for relief, I visit an anesthesiologist at a Kalamazoo pain clinic who performs occipital (near the base of the skull) nerve blocks and trigger point injections, followed by an intravenous lidocaine drip while I am hooked up to an EKG to monitor my heart. Oh, the possible side effects. This drug is a cardiac antiarrhythmic agent, so this is strictly off-label. My nurse friend Sandi rides along as my advocate and monitors the PQRS squiggles while I stare at the defibrillator so conveniently attached to the wall beside me. It is a Medtronic model. How reassuring.

On the ride home, a brainstorm rolls in, and I decide that this prescription does not warrant a refill.

chapter 11

Pick Your Poison

Fear not death, for the sooner we die the longer we will be immortal.
—Ben Franklin[15]

Amen, Ben.
—Susan P. Ryan

Without the slightest improvement under the scheme of enhanced hormonal manipulation, I return to the predictable estradiol patch and schedule an appointment at the Michigan Headache and Neurological Institute in Ann Arbor. It is hard to feel optimism when the last experience left me deflated, but I am still in need of relief. I want to live more fully in retirement instead of scheduling my life around doctors' appointments and cancellations of fun due to migraine.

After hearing of my prior treatment failures, Dr. G suggests DHE 45® (dihydroergotamine) intravenous, and/or Methergine® (methylergonovine) oral, which is used to treat uterine bleeding after childbirth. The possible side effects from ergots of retroperitoneal fibrosis and kidney failure are not on my bucket list. *Severe headache* is a more common side effect. I already have this down pat without consuming the suggested fungus. And ergotamine is contraindicated for Raynaud's patients due to reduced blood flow to limbs. It is another contrarian treatment: what does not kill you makes you stronger. Though the ergots are touted with a 75 percent cure rate for severe migraine, I refuse this scary treatment and pick door number two, Amerge® (naratriptan), a newer triptan to abort migraine. I also begin Anaprox® (naproxen), a prescription-strength anti-inflammatory for ten days, then as needed for up to three days per week. This tears up my gut and MHNI offers me an alternative of Toradol 30mg intramuscular injection as needed for headache. I have used this drug before. It is difficult to self-administer, provides moderate temporary relief of pain without symptoms of nausea, dizziness, and brain fog, so I use it when my other options are exhausted. It takes the edge off my pain but does not erase it. I start Robaxin® 500mg (methocarbamol), a muscle relaxer: 1-2 tablets three times daily as needed. A single tab nails me to the bed whenever headache pain outweighs my need to be upright and feigning functionality. Phenergan® (promethazine) suppositories are prescribed for nausea; they minimize queasiness and vomiting and lessen head pain a few ounces. Or grams if I am in a metric state of mind. Although doctors request patients to rate their pain on a numerical scale, which I dutifully mark on my headache calendar as a reluctant rule-follower, but as someone who enjoys cooking and once compounded pharmaceuticals, I prefer thinking of weight and volume for measuring my pain. It is a perhaps a silly way for me to address chronic pain and it may be my coping strategy. I do not share my pain-rating system with the neurologists; they may refer me to a shrink, and I do not want to spend my time and energy visiting another specialist.

And once again I am back on the brain-train drug gabapentin 100mg each morning, noon, and 200mg at bedtime. I become zombie-like on this med. When I complain of side effects, I am referred to a psychologist at MHNI who prescribes a lower level of exercise than my usual cycling and walking 18 holes on the golf course. Dr. B says "Keep your exertion constant and increase slightly each week. Use a pulse rate monitor to stay in a good range. Make a written plan each evening for the next day. Set a timer to accomplish set times for tasks. Practice yoga breathing." This advice from a wedded-to-the-desk consultant may be good strategy for someone else. Doc does not understand my enthusiasm for sports and exercise. My body requires a certain amount of exercise to sleep through the night and I am not compliant with this order.

September, *nine headache days*. Another normal MRI on 9/14 while side effects from polypharmacy persist. Is this my newest norm? October, *eleven headache days*. I begin ingesting antacids to deal with gastrointestinal wear and tear from prescribed treatments. At the next MHNI visit, gabapentin is increased to 400mg at lunch. Major dizziness. My activities are reduced to knitting scarves and hats on the sofa and reading in between naps. My standard poodle does not understand the disappearance of her daily three-mile walks. I increase my magnesium intake. November, *14 headache days.*

As the barometer rocks and rolls, so goes my brain. I live in a paradise that is sometimes my hell. But I realize that there is a silver lining to my misery. I can predict the arrival of weather fronts twelve hours before they land on the shore of Lake Michigan. Shall I pursue a new career in shoreline meteorology? January, *eleven headache days.*

February: Gabapentin increases to 700mg at bedtime. I restrict fluids in the evening since I cannot safely navigate the path from my bed to the bathroom. Shall I wear a helmet or a diaper to bed? On February 23, Doc increases gabapentin to 700mg three times each day. I feel like a wart on a frog, or maybe just the mossy log beneath the frog. I am immobile on this dose. Unable to drive. Unable to walk and talk at the same time. It is dangerous to live alone while on this regimen. I am drowning, searching for a life raft. Does each remedy need to be worse than the malady?

chapter 12

TOXIC TREATMENTS

Poison is in everything, and no thing is without poison. The dosage makes it either a poison or a remedy.
—Paracelsus[16]

My mother points out the danger lurking inside a bulging can of navy beans on the shelf of the local A & P® as we shop for groceries after school in the 1960s. (The Great Atlantic and Pacific Tea Company was founded in 1859 and led the way to modern supermarkets across the United States through its marketing innovations. With increased competition, it declared bankruptcy in 2015 and is out of business.) At home, I open Compton's Encyclopedia© and learn that botulinum toxin produces a serious form of food poisoning as it attaches to nerve endings, causing paralysis and death. Today, Ona Botulinum Toxin Type A, aka Botox®, is touted for wrinkle eradication, lazy eye syndrome, severe spasms in the neck, arm, and hand muscles, profuse underarm sweating, and it was approved in October 2010 for chronic migraine prevention. As a migraineur, which treatment sounds better: boring holes in my throbbing head or rolling the dice with a paralytic agent?

On March 10, 2011, I arrive at the headache clinic feeling desperate for relief. As usual, there is a long wait after my hours-long drive across the state. I doze in the darkened, womb-like waiting room, where each patient sits alone with her thoughts and pain, avoiding conversation and eye contact. No sharing, no networking. Migraine is a solitary affliction. Sometimes it hurts to talk and especially to listen.

"Susan." Her voice penetrates the darkness, and my assigned Florence Nightingale, wearing a pink fleece jacket over her navy scrubs, leads me to a treatment room, where the meat locker temperature jolts me awake. I scan the room for clues to the future, my future without near daily pain and of dreading my next round of incapacitation. I stare with widened eyes as she sets a clattering tray of syringes loaded with poison on a draped table. On the wall a life-sized poster of a woman's head is marked with Xs, showing the physician where to jab, with front and back views. It appears that some serious target shooting goes on in this room. I hug myself, still safe inside a wooly sweater, and as my optimism resurfaces, I begin making plans for headache-free days ahead. After I have read the entire *Wall Street Journal*, a *New Yorker Magazine*, and a long book of short stories, the doctor strides in, humming a tune. Is it from the musical "Annie?" *The sun will come out tomorrow.* He is sipping a steaming cup of water. He must belong to a caffeine-free cult. Flo trails behind with a space heater to keep Doc's trigger fingers warm. Doc discusses the FDA list of possible complications from Botox injections. I sit undaunted, though shivering sans sweater, baring my neck and shoulders, daring the treatment to succeed. I am ready to sign away my rights, anything for the possibility of a fuller life.

"Any questions, Ms. Ryan?"

"Do you have a bit of duct tape in case my eyelids malfunction? It's a long drive home, my seeing-eye canine, Ella FitzPoodle, is only licensed for daylight driving, and it's getting close to sunset."

Doc smiles and continues his litany. "Fallen arches, acne, hemorrhoids, near death experience, and profound nightmares."

"I'll take the profound nightmares," I say. Signing my consent, I absolve the clinic of whatever harm they may inflict. We discuss dosage as dictated by the FDA vs. what was found to be safe and effective during clinical studies at this very headache institute. "Doc let's start with the lowest effective dose. I'd like to see if I have more than just profound nightmares along with diminishing headaches. And I'm sure I'll be paying out of pocket for each toxic microgram since Blue Cross won't cover this treatment even though the FDA approved it a few months ago. Just when did the government and insurance companies begin practicing medicine?"

Doc nods. "Indeed."

I dangle my feet off the edge of the treatment table and Doc stands behind me with his poison darts. I take a few deep breaths and try to relax the nape of my neck as he snaps on gloves and swabs my neck and forehead with icy alcohol. I shiver. *Déjà vu.*

"Are you ready, Susan?"

"Yes." I close my eyes and brace myself.

"Okay, here we go."

He surprises me with a sneak frontal attack, stabbing me a few times between the eyes, along the eyebrows and in vertical lines up and down my forehead and into the hairline. Needles crunch into muscle with more sensation than I expect and the auditory is unnerving.

"Turn around now," he says.

I swing my legs to the other side of the table away from Doc and he penetrates muscles in my shoulders and neck and up into the hairline. My world fades to black after one particularly jarring jab. "Breathe deeper," I hear through a dark, buzzing tunnel. I feel Doc and the nurse, one on each side, holding me on the treatment table. The nurse guides me to a supine position, places a cool cloth on my neck, and offers a sip of water.

"This is the first time someone fainted in my arms. And you slumped so gently," says Doc.

"Well, don't consider yourself special," I say. "You're not the first to catch me in a swoon. Let's get this done. I'll lie face down and try to stay on the gurney."

"Only three more to go," he says.

I grip the edge of the table as he sticks me again, again, and again. I am a guinea pig, a mammalian pincushion. I wonder if I will stop breathing soon, or maybe later, on the drive home. After my blood pressure inches back to its usual 90/55, I am released to the cashier.

"We're going to give you the old rate," says the clerk at the check-out window. "Just $1,070 for today." Old rate for a new treatment? Am I in Oz?

I recite my practiced line. "It's a good thing I already had my fainting spell."

Not a member of the caffeine-free cult, I grab a cup of Earl Grey tea in the lobby, balancing a tender head on an aching neck. $1,070 divided by 32 injections of botulinum toxin is not a bad deal if it works. I would trade my 401K account for a pain-free existence. I return in ninety days for another round of Botox. After a few more treatments, I notice my smoother forehead in the bathroom mirror. Finally, a bonus side effect, but the headaches still lurk. They seem to be a few degrees less painful but are still frequent and life-interrupting with continuing nausea, dizziness, and an inability to speak coherently. *Le mot juste* vanishes during brainstorms. Doc says, "It is early in the process. Give it more time to see if this is effective for you." My fingers are crossed, and I am wearing a bit of bone on a silver chain around my neck.

Update: Since Botox was FDA-approved for treatment of chronic migraine for patients suffering fifteen or more days per month, I have endured the injections every ninety days for several years. I took a break for a few years and have restarted the treatment. I find that my headaches are not significantly reduced in frequency, but the pain level is lower. The mode of action for Botox is blocking transmission of acetylcholine at the neuromuscular junction, causing a reversible chemical denervation of muscle fibers. The resulting numbness seems to decrease the pain intensity of my migraine, but the nausea, dizziness, and aphasia, an inability to articulate, have continued with each episode. I believe that the paralysis of specific muscles is helpful in reducing pain signals, but this is not a cure for me.

Insurance companies are not eager to pay for Botox, even

though it has been approved by the FDA for preventative treatment of chronic migraine. Sometimes it is covered, sometimes not. Though Botox is quite expensive, it may be worth fighting an insurance company and I also discuss "acceptable" coding with the clinic's billing department. I am staying with this time-consuming and uncomfortable treatment since it is somewhat helpful in reducing my brainstorm burden.

March Madness: *twenty-six migraine days*. I am told again that it will take a while for numbness to set in. I believe my nerve endings become overly stimulated from the needling during Botox administration. No one deserves this quality of life. April, *twenty-two headache days*. A frozen shoulder aggravating the neck and head muscles causes a megaton migraine explosion. I begin working with a new massage therapist in South Haven and schedule my first visit with Lea Ke for acupuncture in St. Joseph, Michigan. She is an amazing healer for some people I know, and I look forward to her treatments. But after several months of regular visits, I do not see a lessening of my brainstorms. Ms. Ke tells me it is time to move on. I admire her. Most doctors do not admit failure to their patients.

In June I return to MHNI for Botox injections. Doc writes for Calan® (verapamil) a calcium channel blocker, which relaxes the muscles of the heart and blood vessels, lowering blood pressure. I am once again a poster child for side effects: dizziness, *headache*, slow heart rate, constipation, tiredness, nausea, severe hypotension. Doc reassures me that this is a good choice, since the drug works as a peripheral vasodilator, meaning it will dissipate heat. Good for my heat intolerance, but not for Raynaud's with my icy fingers and toes. He adds as I slink toward the door,

"You may increase gabapentin to 800-1200mg at bedtime for better sleep. I am currently a sleep-walking zombie on a lower dose and can barely muster a fake laugh. But he is serious. May, *twenty migraine days*.

chapter 13

Awakening the Right Brain

I saw the angel and carved until I set him free.
—Michelangelo[17]

On July 3, 2011, I fly from Grand Rapids, Michigan to Rome for my initial two-weeks residency for the Master of Fine Arts in Writing program at Spalding University. I am thrilled with the opportunity to write in this history-laden location, yet worried about balancing brainstorms with creative output. The weather is hotter than advertised, reaching 100 degrees Fahrenheit in Rome for the first week. Thank goodness for icy air conditioning in the hotel, but I am cooked beyond *al dente* pasta during an excursion to the Coliseum and waiting on queue at the Vatican. I miss out on a visit to nearby Trevi Fountain, the underground catacombs, among other opportunities, due to my heat intolerance and migraine proclivity. Rome is a brutal climate for me in mid-summer. I am a weak gladiator. A fellow student catches me by the arm as I stumble on a cobbled stone street, overcome with heat and an inability to sweat. During the second week, our group of about fifty students and faculty moves into *Tenuta Di Spannocchia*, a 700-year-old organic farm near Sienna in Tuscany. We are informed that the thick walls of the buildings will keep us cool without air conditioning. Not true. I take advantage of a steel pool used for watering livestock and plunge in between lectures, dripping in class with a T-shirt and running shorts pulled over my sodden swimsuit. I find relief wherever I can.

In July, I endure *twenty migraine days* despite *nienta vino in Italia*. But I discover gelato, a divine intervention, with its cooling, delectable comfort. I believe every bit of brain freeze is helpful, releasing me with a dose of temporary amnesia. After discovering this tasty distraction, I buy an Italian-made gelato maker as soon as I get home to soothe my soul without side effects. I begin physical therapy for migraine. I visit a podiatrist for new orthotics. Am I missing anything?

August 24, back to MHNI. "Let's taper gabapentin to zero. Use it strictly as an abortive at bedtime. I want to start you on Effexor® (venlafaxine)" Sure. This is a serotonin-norepinephrine reuptake inhibitor (SNRI) which works by restoring a balance of serotonin and norepinephrine in the brain. I do not experience all the listed side effects, *just* nausea, drowsiness, dizziness, dry mouth, constipation, loss of appetite, trouble sleeping, and easy bruising. Doc adds the old opioid standby, Fioricet, to be used alternately with naratriptan at the onset of migraine. August, *twenty migraine days*. Is this the Inferno or merely Purgatorio?

The coding diagnosis from my chart: *Myofascial regional pain syndrome, chronic daily headache, cervicalgia. Tx: Botulinum Toxin A 155 units in 31 trigger point injections—Frontalis, Corrugator, Procerus, Temporalis, Occipitalis, Suboccipitalis, Splenius Capitis, Semispinalis Capitis, Trapezius, and Levator Scapula* (This Latin litany is a flashback to Catholic school in the 1960s; may it be healing.) *with 30-gauge needles. Avoid rubbing injection sites or icing for two days.* Check.

September, *ten headache days*. Did the decrease in frequency result from pharmaceuticals or cooler temperatures? And the answer is: inconclusive. Perhaps the migraine itself was fatigued and took a wee holiday. (There's a concept: Migraine has a life of its own, like an alien parasite in my body.) And why do I consider ten migraine days per month a holiday?

October, *twenty-one headache days*. On October 19, I meet with Dr. Julia, ND for homeopathic and dietary guidance. I begin her prescribed regimen of Niacin, L-Glutamine, and charcoal tablets to mark bowel transit time. Now this is a novel tactic and perhaps an interesting item for a dinner party conversation starter. Niacin, aka Vitamin B-3, helps the digestive tract metabolize food and produce energy. It is vital for the nervous system and can be used in high doses to help lower elevated cholesterol levels. I could use this effect. However, side effects include *headache*, blurred vision, and low blood pressure. Since I already enjoy these symptoms, will they be enhanced? L-Glutamine is used for sickle cell disease, trauma, such as burns and other critical illnesses. It is considered for so-called "leaky gut syndrome" which I have been accused of having by another naturopathic physician, but there are no studies to support this. And possible side effects include nausea, bloating, dizziness, heartburn, and stomach pain. These are currently among my symptoms during migraine and could be caused by some of the other prescribed drugs. I have a low expectation though appreciate the kindness of the practitioner who seems to care, calling twice to check on me.

November, *twenty headache days*. December, *fourteen migraine days*. Merry Christmas. January 2012, *thirteen headache days*. February, *twenty-two migraine days*. Holy Mary, Mother of God! Can it get any worse? There are only six days without my monster this month. Or did I forget to chart a daily occurrence?

Chiropractic adjustment on February 17. On February 22, the MHNI Neurologist issues a script for isometheptene 65mg (a sympathomimetic which causes vasoconstriction, possibly useful for acute headache). It is the active ingredient in Midrin®. Dose: 1-2 capsules up to three times daily as needed for headache. Space four hours apart from Amerge doses. I search for this specialty item at three compounding pharmacies. Good luck with that scavenger hunt.

March, *eight migraine days*; April, *nine days*; May, *fifteen days*. I am instructed to increase the melatonin dose at bedtime and add Zanaflex® (tizanidine), two-three tablets of this muscle relaxer at bedtime. The usual side effects hit me, including dry mouth, dizziness, lightheadedness, constipation, weakness, tiredness. Sounds redundant, but I experience each one again. I also have the so-called serious side effects of fainting, slow heart rate, and hallucinations. Scintillating images dance in the air over my bed. It is unnerving. I consider calling 1-800-EXORCIST. And along with these daunting side effects, I still endure debilitating headaches oh-so-freaking-often.

My mother's health takes a nosedive from complications

of diabetes. I begin spending more time at her home, bearing the bullying of her husband Bill, who does not want me there. I try to be helpful without interfering. It is one of the toughest situations I ever encounter. I'll spare the details, but I now realize that this episode may have contributed to my increasing number of migraine days per month. While my mother lost her right leg above the knee, her abusive husband disappeared at the time of her surgery and never called her again. I worked through mom's divorce while she attempted to recover physically and emotionally in her mid-eighties.

On July 18, I travel to Paris for my second residency of the MFA program for two weeks. With seven siblings nearby and Bill out of the house, I still feel a bit guilty for leaving town, but I know that there will be more than enough to do when I return. There is. I hire an attorney for Mom. Bill filed for divorce days after he left. He never spoke to Mom again. Mom's attorney says, "Con men have no age limit or expiration date. I unfortunately see this kind of thing often."

July, *twenty headache days*.

In Paris I write and read my work to fellow writers and participate in round table discussions of each other's work. It is a great respite for me to be so far away from the troubles in Michigan, though my mother is always in my thoughts. I miss an excursion to Monet's home in Giverny, due to migraine, though spend a few hours at the Louvre. Though it is my second visit, I am still awed by the actual art I have enjoyed in books. At Musee d'Orsay I am wowed by Manet; though it is Le Centre Pompidou where Chagall's genius lights me up, and the Rodin Museum, where I find my ultimate happy place. The bronze sculptures arrest me and invite me to sit on a bench and share their company. I feel my late father's presence as I inhale the art. He loved to draw, paint, and sculpt, and I am seeing this magnificent art with his eyes. Upon entering the Chartres Cathedral, I am overcome with tears, hearing of pilgrims who crawled on a labyrinthine pattern in supplication. My mother now has only one knee. She has given up so much in this life. I purchase a blue crystal rosary in the gift shop for her. She is a devout Catholic, who graduated from Marygrove, a Catholic College for women in Detroit prior to marrying and raising eight children. She played organ in church and shared her faith with her family.

At the Palace of Versailles, I remember stories my father told of camping on these historic grounds in winter during WWII. I imagine him in his early twenties, sipping champagne during his time off, and beginning his lifelong habit of sketching what he saw, including a young French woman named Eve. My sister Patti has this charcoal sketch. Despite the burden of headache, I absorb much through traveling with a bit of time for reflection. I am grateful that I took advantage of the chance to do my semester residencies abroad. Though I missed out on some opportunities when I felt too ill to participate, it was more enlightening than studying at home. The brainstorms would have happened with or without my change of scenery. I just did my best to eat well, hydrate adequately, and prioritize sleep in each time zone.

While my mother recovers in between major surgeries, I travel back and forth across the state from South Haven to Ann Arbor. I hate to complain about another sinus infection during this time, but it negatively impacts my sleep, energy level, decision-making abilities, and migraine frequency and intensity. August, *thirteen* headache days; September, *ten days;* October, *ten days.*

Appointments continue in Ann Arbor including relaxation technique coaching with a staff psychologist who does guided imagery for hand-warming. My hands are nearly always cold since I developed Raynaud's after taking a prescription migraine remedy. Doc says, "Imagine drawing blood into your hands, which warms the extremities, and pulls blood away from swollen cerebral arteries." I am prescribed doxycycline, a broad-spectrum antibiotic used in the treatment of infections caused by bacteria and parasites, for a few weeks. What are these brain pain gurus thinking? This tough on the gut drug is used for Lyme Disease. I unearth a study suggesting the "Use of Doxycycline with Triptan to Determine Effects of Neuroinflammatory Markers in the Brain." This regimen gives me a week of diarrhea after killing off my gut microbiome. Again. This guinea pig survives and awaits her next experiment.

November, *nine headache days*; December, *nine headaches*; January 2013, *thirteen headache days.* My gut is complaining and competing with my head for attention with the side effects of off-the-wall treatments taking a toll on my GI tract. On February 26, I visit with a gastroenterologist who discontinues magnesium, CoQ10, (an antioxidant produced by the body and commonly prescribed as a supplement, thought to decrease migraine and improve cardiovascular function) and oral anti-inflammatories. "No more NSAIDs for you," Doc Z says. "You have developed an ulcer." I begin a proton-pump inhibitor for thirty days to protect my ravaged gastric mucosa. I try to adhere to a restrictive

FODMAP diet, which is Fermentable Oligosaccharides, Disaccharides, Monosaccharides, and short chain Polyols, all sugars that the small intestine poorly absorbs. No more milk, wheat, beans, artichokes, asparagus, onion, garlic, apples, cherries, peaches, pears, oh my! I take extra doses of Citrucel, and a probiotic.

February, *fifteen headache days*; March, *thirteen headache days*; April, *nine headache days*.

Dr. G moves to Texas, and I meet a new neurologist at MHNI who starts me on Calan® (verapamil), a calcium channel blocker twice daily. Labeled uses: high blood pressure, angina, tachycardia. I experience dizziness upon standing and especially in the shower with my eyes closed. Doc P considers me for a vagal nerve stimulation study, but I am turned down for some reason. Probably too dizzy and hypotensive.

May, *sixteen headache days*. Gabapentin is increased to 400mg at bedtime and 100mg three times during the day. How will I drive a car through the ensuing brain fog? I flash back to a long ago visit to Space Mountain at Disney and a rollercoaster ride in the dark. My body does not know what is coming; I am just along for the wild, unpredictable ride.

June, *twenty headache days*. I take another steroid burst to break up near-daily headaches, and it is suggested that I start on either Prozac® (fluoxetine) or Lexapro® (escitalopram) for migraine prevention with fewer anticholinergic effects. I speak with a Walgreen pharmacist, and he agrees with me that I should not take this class of drug with a triptan, which is the only drug that provides any escape from migraine. The worry is serotonin syndrome, something to be avoided. According to Medline, an online resource for medical professionals, early symptoms include "tremors, dizziness, and headache." This may progress to "hypertension, rapid heart rate, loss of muscle coordination," and can become *life-threatening* with "high fever, tremor, seizures, irregular heartbeat, and unconsciousness," says the Mayo Clinic website. High levels of serum serotonin can occur with the administration of a drug like an SSRI given with a triptan. Caffeine may also trigger an episode. Side effects are real and need to be monitored.

On July 3, I fly from Chicago to Dublin for my third residency in the MFA program. My room at Trinity College is unairconditioned and Our Lady of Perpetual Heat is also in residence. Perhaps I should not make a Catholic joke at a Protestant College, but as an Irish American lass, what the hell, since it is not possible to dial down the building's thermostat. Why is normally cool Ireland experiencing a hellish heat wave? With windows open, the sounds of revelry from the pub below travel to my room every night for the first week. I plug my ears and bury my head beneath pillows while wishing for a sleety storm. I long for a bucket of ice to soothe my pain. My Irish eyes are weeping. I awaken to my favorite comfort food each bleary-eyed morning: Irish soda bread with Irish butter and tea, but each night delivers a hot, daunting din.

The second week our group travels across the Emerald Isle to the west coast. Galway is quieter and cooler. A side trip to the Aran Island of Inishmore is worth all the headaches of the past week in Dublin. Cycling through sheep traffic jams, swimming in the refreshing Irish Sea with non-poisonous moon jellyfish, and hiking to the edge of the sea cliffs of Inis Mor, the beauty sublimates my pain. During my third week in Ireland, a friend from Michigan joins me. Since I am the designated driver with prior experience in left hand drive, I power through a tour of the west and the south coasts. While I pop triptans and acetominophen, we travel unscathed, dodging carloads of oncoming tourists and meandering sheep. St. Patrick is looking out for us. The clockwise round-abouts are a wee challenge as I ask my co-pilot to designate an exit path before we enter the pattern. "Give me a nine, twelve, or three o'clock cue, or prepare for another round trip." My copilot closes his eyes, and I rely on my Irish instinct while negotiating the narrow roads clogged with summer traffic. The signs blur by in long, drawn-out Gaelic with small English subtitles below as if an afterthought, so tough to read from an inside lane. I am sober, sort of. Under the influence of migraine is not optimal for an American attempting left side driving and may be equivalent to imbibing a pint or two of Guinness™ at lunch. Who knows, but some medical investigator could devise a prospective randomized study to consider impairment by migraine versus the drink. I meet this challenge and survive. But I feel the anxiety of my poor passenger, a former Marine who served in Vietnam. I should have warned him about "passenger in the ditch." This tip is offered to Americans as they pick up rental cars in Ireland. Most vehicles are heavily scarred on the passenger side from contact with brambles, and many side mirrors disappear into the brush during tourist travels on the Emerald Isle. July, *nineteen headache days.*

chapter 14

IMPATIENT INPATIENT

When many remedies are proposed for a disease,
it means the disease is incurable.
—Leon Tolstoy[18]

A rebounding, pounding migraine fires continuously during my three-week trip to Ireland for graduate school. While I try to enjoy the land of my ancestors, summer heat scorches my sensitive brain and the migraine reblooms each day. 'Tis Bloomsday in Ireland where we celebrate the life of James Joyce, but as soon as my holiday is over, I am hospitalized at a renowned headache institute in the Midwest with the diagnosis of medication overuse headache (MOH). My daily use of a triptan, a vasoconstrictor, which works on the blood vessels and nerve endings in the brain is the culprit, along with acetaminophen. No Guinness. No Irish Whiskey. No opioids. Just Imitrex. As soon as each dose wears off, a fresh migraine creeps in.

What brings me to this point? *When does acute migraine become chronic migraine? When it is no longer cute.* What starts as a monthly brainstorm becomes my way of life. By breaching the threshold of fifteen migraine days per month for at least three months, I vault into the chronic category. What fresh hell is this? From one or three to seventeen per month in a matter of years, this is likely caused by my determination to work through migraine as if it does not exist. Am I in denial, or do I have Wonder Woman complex, thinking I can overcome anything? I pop ibuprofen, naproxen, aspirin, acetaminophen, and lots of prescription drugs as I battle my demon. The brain change, called neuroplasticity, is a remodeling of the neurons, where these cells become more sensitive, more reactive, and accustomed to the flow of chemicals I ingest to tamp down pain. As soon as the blood level of medication drops below an effective concentration, neurons light up complaining, "we want more." This reminds me of Audrey, the man-eating plant in *The Little Shop of Horrors*.[19] Audrey's mantra was "feed me." And she was thirsting for blood.

Could I have avoided this life sentence of chronic migraine? Perhaps. A genetic component turns on the pain pathway when I enter puberty and experience my first brainstorm. Bathed in hormones at fluctuating levels, my sensitive brain is primed for pain at age twelve. If I had lain in bed each month for a few days with ice on my noggin and a hot water bottle on my cramping belly, would I be headache-free after menopause when hormones take their sabbatical? It is not possible to study this supposition without an identical twin as a control. My theoretical twin would embrace her monthly pain, riding it out on the couch, eschewing modern medicine, while lacking the drive to take on the world and all it has to offer. Will her headaches eventually subside? Alas I have no twin, no control for a lifestyle experiment. Is my chronic migraine caused by ambition, my Type A+ personality? Maybe. Neuroplasticity is a rewiring of the brain provoked by environmental and psychological cues. I never give my brain a chance to adapt to monthly headaches while I do my utmost to tamp down pain and carry on. Pathways form to facilitate pain. Pain begets pain and it becomes my default setting.

At sixteen when I begin working in a drugstore, assisting the pharmacists, I learn about "better living through chemistry." Whenever I dare to call in sick, the pharmacists offer cures: tetracycline for a sore throat, salves and ace bandages for sports injuries, and analgesics for pain. No need for down time. During this apprenticeship I am gob smacked to find that tiny pills can do so much for a body. They contain doses of magic. During high school I decide to become a pharmacist and own a corner drugstore with a soda fountain. But that is a story for another book.

Meanwhile, in the summer of 2013, I check into the Headache Hotel and submit to their cure. The Eagles song *Hotel California* plays in my head. I feel vulnerable, alone, and wonder if I will ever leave. I am carrying a head full of pain that has not eased up in over a month. I cross two state lines in search of relief, anticipating a thirty-minute office consultation with a headache specialty neurologist following a ninety-minute wait. I carry my headache journals and *Migraine*, a book by neurologist and fellow migraineur, Oliver Sacks, M.D. I expect to drive home with a cup of caffeine and a few new prescriptions. Instead, I am instructed to proceed to inpatient admission at St. Hildegard Hospital. Do not pass Go. Do not collect any triptans. "Expect to stay for a week or more," I am told. While the headache experts sort out my complaining brain, I will detox from the current stew of ineffective pharmaceuticals. The neurologists recommend a "six-week drug holiday from triptans, withdrawing safely over six to ten days as an inpatient." I am not ready for this interruption of my life, but what life?

Check-in time is in two hours, so I visit a nearby REI store to pick up some patient-casual attire for my new role as inpatient. This may be interesting, I think. As a science major in college, I love lab testing, experimenting, and checking out hypotheses. But I would prefer to observe the patient rather than inhabit her.

Upon admission I am offered a "one time dose" of Dolophine® (methadone) 10mg with Phenergan® (promethazine) 50mg intravenously. *Mainlining.* I am shocked at both the route of administration and the choice of drugs. Methadone is used for heroin withdrawal and in maintenance treatment for opioid addicts. Am I a triptan junkie? Promethazine is an anti-nausea and sedative-effect drug with side effects listed of **tissue necrosis and gangrene with IV use.** I decline this happy hour special. The nurse seems surprised. Do most patients take this bait? Without a nearby advocate, I do not choose to be unconscious. The afternoon nurse lights me up with an IVP (intravenous push) of 80mg of Depo Medrol® (methylprednisolone). I suppose that the intent of this steroid is to mitigate the detox process while my brain drains its current load of drugs so the docs can refill the resulting vacuum with a combo of rave new cures. My usual 90/60 blood pressure inches up to 110/62. I am on high alert as I assess my ability to endure the medical team's plan.

My hospital orders include magnesium sulfate IV; Benadryl® (diphenhydramine) IV, an antihistamine which may be used for motion sickness and some movement disorders like Parkinson's; Norflex® (orphenadrine citrate) IV, a muscle relaxer; Toradol (ketorolac tromethamine) IV, a nonsteroidal anti-inflammatory; Depacon® (valproic acid) IV, an antiepileptic with a common side effect of *headache*. Really. Surprised at the IV route for my PRN (as needed) meds, I realize that this may be justification for insurance coverage of my inpatient stay, since I cannot self-administer these treatments via IV at home. On the third hospital day, the IV site in my left-hand blows, and a nurse relocates the catheter a few inches up on top of my wrist. My veins burn with each dose and bruises blossom. I beg for oral or intramuscular meds but am refused.

I am weaned off gabapentin, an anticonvulsant and nerve pain drug, and started on Vivactil® (protriptyline), a tricyclic antidepressant, and Nimotop® (nimodipine), a calcium channel blocker used to reduce blood pressure during brain bleeds. Now this is a serious indication, and I wonder how it may affect my lower-than-normal blood pressure. I am not optimistic about this "triptan-free drug holiday," considering the side effects of so many heavy-artillery off-label drugs. I remember studying the myriad problems with "polypharmacy" patients during a hospital internship and now I am living it. If I maintain my wits, I may survive this experiment. I sleep with one eye open if I sleep at all in this place.

The first night in the hospital is rough. I worry. I wonder; did

I make the right choice in coming here? Since I noticed no real progress at MHNI, I thought it may be time for a reboot, but did I make a mistake in revisiting this clinic? Here in the hospital, I feel I am losing control, and it scares me. I receive Toradol IV at 10 pm along with my requested icepack for my throbbing head. The staff initially brings me a hot pack, contrarian treatment for a volcano, my exploding cranium, although the heat might be sweet on a stiff neck. At 3 am a nurse pushes Benadryl IV. I sleep heavily drugged until 7 am, when I awaken with a Sahara-dry mouth, wondering where I am, until a scrum of MDs and PAs enters my room on their rounds. From the bottom of a well, I hear myself questioning the whitecoats about their medication choices and I am told, "It's protocol." Not one of them touches me, looks into my eyes, or answers my very specific questions. They exit in a white wave and close the door so they can discuss me in the hallway without hearing from me.

After breakfast I attend an orientation to the program, a biofeedback session, a nutrition lecture, and a coping skills class. I listen through a pea-soup fog, my migraine clanging from a distance like a lighthouse warning. The headache is ever-present, but I am not. A cocktail of new drugs has moved in and taken me off to the side as an observer. I feel dislocated from pain while observing from outside of my body. Is it really me who is living in this state, or am I starring in a B-movie? I begin Depakote® 500mg (divalproex sodium, an anti-seizure medication) IVPB (intravenous piggyback) with a liter bag of saline as chaser every twelve hours for three days. I rely on topical ice for pain control. It is the only thing that makes any difference. Pleased that I have not yet been frostbitten, I put up with the only side effect: wet pajamas from a leaky Ziplock™ bag. I guess they do not stock frozen peas or a sealed ice pack in this place.

The next day T.S. treats me with acupuncture at trigger points, spawning a monstrous bruise on my left sternocleidomastoid, which morphs into a giant hickey. I might be embarrassed if I felt well enough. While brushing my teeth the next day I am shocked to see the *aubergine*-colored beauty in the mirror. My eyes are dry and fuzzy, but this Dracula love bite is not something to overlook. During prior acupuncture treatments, I experienced a few episodes of minor bleeding upon removal of needles, but this is the ugliest stigmata yet. I decline a future visit from this individual. He may go for the jugular next time. I sign up for a visit with physical therapist Sylvia, for some gentle stretching of my neck and shoulders.

July 31, Depo Medrol (steroid) IM at 11pm. I feel better for a few hours, but I wonder why the medical geniuses inject something that keeps me awake at bedtime? How about a morning dose? Sleep should be high priority for healing. My new oral meds: protriptyline, a tricyclic antidepressant "to be used under close supervision," according to the package insert, gives me side effects of insomnia, low blood pressure, and numbness of extremities; Nimotop® (Nimodipine), a calcium-channel blocker originally developed for hypertension, but is more often used for treatment of subarachnoid hemorrhage, a form of cerebral bleeding. Is my brain bleeding? This drug lowers my already low blood pressure to a dangerous level. I have trouble getting up from bed without collapsing and I cannot remember to push the call button whenever I head for the bathroom. If I hit my head due to drug-induced hypotension, perhaps the brain bleed drug may be warranted.

The seventh floor of St. Hildegard Hospital is reserved for headache clinic inpatients. On my second day in the hospital, I venture out of my room for physical therapy, biofeedback, and into the patient lounge for a group therapy session. Most of the patients are women, with a few men in the mix, battling brain injury, migraine, and cluster headache. I meet a patient with a dented, scarred head, another with an inoperable brain tumor, a few with concomitant seizures. Several sport PICC lines (a peripherally inserted central catheter), a form of IV access for administration of substances that should not be administered peripherally. After enduring a few days of searing peripheral IVs, I understand why so many of the long-term inpatients have graduated to PICC lines. Their veins have collapsed from caustic infusions. There is a teenage girl who traveled weeks ago from Germany with her mother as her advocate for headache treatment. Every person is here because her life is not her own. It belongs to misery. A few patients have been here for over a month. A recreational therapist encourages group participation and offers hand and scalp massage. Two women complain that their hair is too tender to be touched. I feel blessed to be (in my mind) the healthiest patient on the floor. I do my best to cheer up others, sharing a few goodies I pick up on forays to the hospital gift shop. Though I am nauseous, in pain, dizzy, and bored, I am better off than many of the others. I feel like a poseur. Perhaps I should relinquish my spot to someone who really needs it.

It is summer outside the window of the hospital. The view teases me with a golf driving range and Lake Michigan two blocks away. I am not allowed to leave the building without a hospital employee, so I latch onto Kate, a Recreation Therapist who escorts a few mobile patients for an amble around the block. This dear woman saves my sanity with a couple of absorbing books that keep me in bed for a few days while the questionable course continues. With ice on my head, I read *Devil in the White City* by Erik Larson. This historical non-fiction book takes place during the 1893 World's Fair. Alternate chapters switch to a concomitant story of possibly the world's first modern serial killer, (a medical doctor!) running rampant in Chicago. I wonder if any of his victims were murdered nearby as I try to ignore the burning in my veins from "treatments." Both of my hands are puffed and bruised, and the IV sites are relocated in incremental moves up my arms while I continue to request oral or intramuscular meds. It feels bizarre to be held in a hospital, almost without a choice. I must be desperate for relief to submit to this iffy situation. Many of the patients are so spaced out. They stare blankly instead of answering my friendly questions. The physicians and their PAs are in a hurry to get in and out of my room during morning rounds while I ask "too many questions" about my care. I make suggestions, refuse some of their counterintuitive treatments, and the medical staff seem annoyed when I ask for the reasoning behind their drug choices. "This is our protocol," they say each time. One size apparently will be made to fit all. And I am labeled a difficult patient.

On August 3, I leave the floor with Kate, RT, attending a jazz piano concert on another floor. She introduces me to a 102-year-old woman who has forgotten her hearing aids at home a few blocks away. Phyllis wears a hospital-provided portable amplifier to enjoy the music. She is an inspiration, and I wonder if she ever has migraine. Probably not. I believe the human brain is not equipped to withstand this type of assault for that many decades. I find it sweet to taste freedom for an hour. Before heading back to my room, I stop in the café for a steaming cup of forbidden fruit: French Roast Caribou Coffee® and a bag of peanuts. What a party after being restricted to one Lipton® teabag per day, rationed by the nurses on my floor. It may be against doctors' orders, but WTF. I am a patient, not a prisoner, or so I tell myself. And I feel better for a while with the oh-so-slight caffeine buzz.

I try to stay active while in the hospital, but it is difficult while tethered to an IV pole. I ride a rickety, whining exercise bike in the patient lounge, followed by an ice pack on the head, reclining once again in bed. Patients on this unit are submissive: ready and willing to accept whatever the docs deem essential treatment. Out of desperation, we are human guinea pigs, lab rats.

I am discharged from the hospital on August 5. Either my insurance company has pulled the plug, or the neurologists have run out of options. I do not feel any better; I think I am worse. But I am eager to leave this failed experiment. Though starring in an uncomfortable dream, burdened with pain, I now feel less concern. I am resigned to this state as my new normal. But it is time to return to the safety of home since there are no cures on the horizon from this vantage point. I wave off all sedating drugs such as muscle relaxers and antihistamines for twelve hours before discharge so I can negotiate the drive home. Stopping in the cafeteria on my way out, I fortify my weakened self with a chicken sandwich and a cup of nectar: black coffee. Over lunch I psych myself to prepare for the 120-mile drive around the bottom of Lake Michigan. I find my dusty car in the hospital parking garage and embark on a white-knuckled journey, driving 45 mph in the right lane of the Dan Ryan Expressway, praying to get out of the city before rush hour. I stop at Walgreen in my hometown of South Haven, Michigan and drop off a sheaf of new prescriptions. The technician informs me that half of the items are not stocked. My meds are too exotic for this resort village.

The pharmacist calls an hour later and says, "I'm worried about you. Before I fill these scripts, I want you to visit with your primary care doctor. You two can figure out what may be necessary. But I don't recommend that you take all these meds at the same time." Amen, my RPh guardian angel.

And thank goodness for Ruth, my primary care PA in South Haven. She spends an hour going over the newly prescribed drugs, and we debate the pros and cons of each one and how it could possibly tame my headaches without killing me. I start on:

1. Lioresal® (baclofen), indicated for muscle spasm from MS and spinal cord injuries.

2. Migranal® Nasal Spray (dihydroergotamine), an ergot alkaloid (from a fungus). It acts as a heavy-duty vasoconstrictor that blows the top off my volcano, after initiating a new biting pain behind my eyes with the first whiff.

3. Gabapentin (again) indicated for nerve pain and epilepsy (so mind-numbing).

4. Ketorolac (again), an NSAID which strafes my stomach lining even with the concomitant—

5. Prilosec® (omeprazole), a proton-pump inhibitor for ulcers with side effects of dementia, increased risk of osteoporosis, and decreased magnesium absorption. I find it puzzling to take this drug just to tolerate the side effects of the NSAID. It interferes with magnesium absorption which my brain so greatly needs according to headache experts.

6. Nimodipine, a calcium channel blocker which relaxes blood vessels and lowers blood pressure.

7. Protriptyline, a tricyclic antidepressant; The headache docs call it "activating" as opposed to sedating. Being awake all night is the last thing I need. Why is this part of the protocol?

8. Zanaflex ® (tizanidine), a skeletal muscle relaxant, for Lou Gehrig's, cerebral palsy, dystonia, and contraindicated for low blood pressure, my usual status.

After two weeks at home, my headache frequency is not diminished and the side effects mount. At my next office visit, the PA at the Headache Clinic prescribes:

9. Cymbalta® (duloxetine), a selective serotonin and norepinephrine reuptake inhibitor antidepressant. The package insert says that "Duloxetine affects chemicals in the brain that may be unbalanced in people with depression." Hell, I am not depressed, I am pissed-off. Maybe this is the distraction I need to forget that I have a migraine every stinking day. And then she adds the scariest drug of all:

10. Zyprexa® (olanzipine), an antipsychotic medication that affects chemicals in the brain. It is used to treat schizophrenia and bipolar disorder. The drug comes with a BLACK BOX WARNING: "Zyprexa may impair your thinking or reactions. Be careful if you drive or do anything that requires you to be alert. May cause high cholesterol, high blood pressure, high blood sugar, exercise intolerance . . ." and more. After a single dose, I decide not to comply with this order. It sounds like an early death sentence. I would prefer something more expeditious such as hemlock.

At last, I am rewarded with a triptan,

11. Imitrex® (sumatriptan) IM injection. Alleluia. What a novel idea to offer something that may relieve my migraine, is FDA approved for this purpose, and only hurts when I stab my quadriceps with the needle. But why not oral? I suppose that the thinking of the neuro guru is that if I really want it, I may think twice about

using the needle. Let us make this difficult so you do not overuse it again. Compliance would be easy if only I had less than three headache days each week.

After the Neurology PA complains about my noncompliance, my refusal to follow some of the frightening and harmful orders from this clinic, I ask if she suffers from chronic migraine. She does not respond. I know it is difficult to understand a day in the life of a migraineur from the outside. But whenever I meet a doctor or nurse who has experienced some of my symptoms, she earns credibility. She comes to work with migraine, experiences myriad side effects from so-called treatments, all while enduring pain, nausea, dizziness, vomiting, and a real difficulty in articulating her thoughts. Unless you have experienced the pain and hangover a migraineur feels, it is difficult to understand what your patient needs. Like alcoholism treatment, many of the doctors and therapists who treat these patients are often in recovery themselves. One size does not fit all, though it seems that this renowned clinic has a checklist of drugs and treatments for all patients regardless of their phenotype. Their strategy did not work for me, and I wonder if my fellow zombie patients have been released from their pain and lengthy hospitalizations. I hope so.

Shortly after this episode, I return to the Michigan Headache and Neurological Institute in Ann Arbor for my continuing headache management. The staff are reasonable and not eager to subject me to hospitalization, though they have an inpatient option. I understand that there are few drugs available to treat chronic migraine that are FDA approved for this indication. Brain drugs for other purposes are fair game since the actual cause is difficult to pinpoint. It is all in the head. The sensitive migraine brain does not reveal its secrets on MRI scans, EEG tracings, or X-rays, unless a tumor is present.

August, *twenty-one headache days*, mostly in a druggy fog. On August 19, I begin another steroid burst to break up the continuing brainstorm. I sip antacid Mylanta® (aluminum/magnesium hydroxide/simethicone) with the steroids to assuage a blooming ulcer from the onslaught of drugs. I add Prilosec twice a day. September, *sixteen headache days*. It was the summer of fog and pain. May autumn be better.

chapter 15

IN NEED OF NEEDLING

Your brain has the power to modify your pain perception.
—Wim Hof[20]

October 10, 2014, my first visit with Dr. Sobor, an M.D. who specializes in pain management. I am amazed to find such a specialized practitioner in the small town of South Haven who becomes the fourth acupuncturist to pierce my skin. He starts by placing a dozen or so fine needles into the traditional sites for headache. "Just relax, Susan," he says while I willingly become the victim of a planned porcupine attack. After I am trapped like a frog pinned onto a dissecting tray, Doc dims the lights and leaves the room. I am not yet feeling the suggested relaxation and move on to intentional yoga breathing, saying R-E-L-A-X as my mantra with each long exhale until I nearly pass out. After twenty minutes he returns and drills me with trigger point injections in the temporomandibular joint of the jaw (TMJ) and trapezius, a pair of trapezoid-shaped muscles which extend from the occipital bone at the base of the skull to the lower thoracic vertebrae of the spine and across to the scapula-—collar bones. It may be worthwhile to revisit this fellow since I sleep well for the next four nights without any interruption by headache. Sleep is my best medicine when I can get it.

Once again, I use Imitrex to abort headaches, but by injection only. I know too well how triptans, when used more than two or three days per week, cause rebound migraine, but my life has become a continuous resounding, rebounding headache. My other weapons are stomach searing NSAIDS or acetaminophen with minimal pain diminishment and a propensity to cause rebound like the triptans if consumed more than two or three days a week. Quality of life is not an issue any one of my physicians has discussed with me. Their instruction is either "increase the dosage" or "add this drug." But Dr. Sobor is not writing prescriptions for me. He asks me where it hurts and how I suffer; he asks about my lifestyle and seems genuinely concerned with healing. His therapy is unique, treating the patient holistically. I try to believe him when he says, **"I will cure you."**

On October 15, I return to see Dr. Sobor. He prescribes moist heat twice daily over the kidneys and adrenal glands. He calls it an "energy treatment for my adrenal fatigue." Sure. Stress will fatigue one's adrenals, the source of cortisol, a stress hormone. He taps needles into my legs and back. While I am full of needles, we discuss his art. He creates huge metallic sculptures as a hobby. I suggest a porcupine for his next subject. Afterward I head to a local spa and relax on a heated table while enjoying a facial treatment at 10:30. I attempt to practice self-care, something that I often overlook, while immersed in a busy career or overwhelmed by chronic pain. I feel fine-oh-fine after this indulgence until the barometer plunges in the afternoon, and a migraine blooms at 2:45. My rosy glow pales as a brainstorm rages.

October 17, Dr. Sobor injects deep into my Trapezius muscles with lidocaine 0.1 percent. On October 18, I bicycle 25 miles. Twenty-four hours later a headache roars. Rats. On October 21, I receive more energy packs and Raynaud's needled treatments for my icy fingers and toes. October 24, acupuncture for migraine, and trapezius release with lidocaine injections. The injection sites feel very sore, but I enjoy the hot packs after treatment to left forehead and eyebrow area. I try sleeping on a doctor recommended TempurPedic™ pillow. It smells funny and gives me a stiff neck.

On October 26, it's early to bed and I awake with hallucinations and dizziness. I decrease the bedtime Tizanidine dose (muscle relaxer). Though Dr. Sobor does not write any prescriptions for me, nor intervenes in dosage adjustments of neurologist-prescribed pharmaceuticals, he listens to my complaints of drug side effects. October 27, more hallucinations, dizziness, and a migraine. October 28, I am awakening too often in the middle of the night, so I begin tapering off protriptyline, a tricyclic antidepressant with activating effects. I read that this drug is used off-label for narcolepsy. Duh. Which genius thinks this is a proper treatment for a patient who has been suffering with insomnia? October, *nineteen headache days*; November, *thirteen days;* December, *ten days.*

January 7, 2015, I pass out during trigger point injections.

Dr. Sobor appears excited to witness this, calling it "a remarkable turning point in [my] recovery." I am not overly impressed since I am skilled at passing out. Some of my childhood memories are of fainting during Mass on warm Sunday mornings and waking up slung over my father's shoulder while being carried outdoors. I fainted at times after my weekly allergy shots during grade school. Since my vasovagal response is impressive, I do not understand how passing out is indicative of a breakthrough, but I listen to Dr. Sobor and try to believe in his belief. How often I have fallen for my healers and their promises of a cure. But I have become one of little faith after so many disappointments. Today I will settle for reducing the headache frequency to a manageable level, with a dull roar instead of a hurricane. There have been other medical professionals who have touted their ability to heal me without success, and now my Pollyanna veneer is worn down to the thickness of a single molecule. My nerve cells burn through any treatment prescribed to date.

January 9, occipital trigger point injections to release tension. This seems counter-intuitive as my muscles tense up at the very thought of menacing needles penetrating muscles near the base of my skull. January 16, more energy treatments with electrodes attached to acupuncture needles. I am the body electric. (Apologies to Walt Whitman.) January, *sixteen headache days.*

February 3, Dr. Sobor administers trigger point injections to my overly sensitive face for sinusitis and migraine. Maximal OUCHY. I want to kick him. February 6, acupuncture treatment. February 10, another round of the antibiotic Augmentin from my primary care PA for another sinus infection. February 26, office visit with ear, nose, and throat specialist, Dr. Strabbing.

After viewing my CAT scan he says, "There is nothing I can surgically repair, but I can squirt lidocaine up your sinuses for temporary relief." No thank you. Achoo. He refers me to Dr. Charleston at the University of Michigan Adult Neuropathic and Head Pain Clinic. During residency these two physicians had worked together on clinical studies and authored a paper on this technique they call "sphenopalatine nerve block." I would like to watch another patient undergo this treatment before I submit to it. February, *sixteen headache days*. I do not like this pattern. I do not like you Mr. Grinch. Your treatments scare and your needles pinch. (No reflection on Dr. Charleston or Dr. Strabbing. They are decent fellows. And an apology to the late, great Dr. Seuss.)

I am icing my head at bedtime in the middle of winter in my drafty house by the lake. An electric pad on the foot of my bed thaws my blue toes. Ice on the head works better than any drug, but it only provides temporary relief. I consume omeprazole to protect my complaining gut. I discontinue the asthma/allergy drug Singular® (montelukast) after the allergy season. I am told by one of my healers, "Your mast cells and immune system are wiped out." I believe so. The prescribed chemicals are not improving my life in any way. I also DC Nasocort® (triamcinolone acetonide) nasal spray and taper off progesterone, estrogen, and gabapentin. Again. Again. And again.

March 16, I take a sublingual homeopathic remedy provided by Grassflower, R.N. Yes, that is her full legal name. The sugar pills containing a few molecules of what my migraine is asking for is an awesome cure. I awake on 3/17 without pain and increased energy. I love this placebo effect. It is St. Patrick's Day, and I celebrate with a single Guinness. March, *only one headache day*. Sláinte! Erin go Brach! Let's toast to the power of placebos or coincidence. But this cure is short-lived and migraine sneaks back, with the frequency and intensity resuming their too-familiar place in my life.

chapter 16

The Frankenstein Treatment

Our greatest human adventure is the evolution of consciousness. We are in this life to enlarge the soul, liberate the spirit, and light up the brain.
—Tom Robbins[21]

Electricity reanimated the dead in Mary Shelley's novel, "Frankenstein."[22] Can a transcutaneous electrical nerve stimulator restore my brain to factory settings? I read in a medical journal about a new treatment for migraine called Cefaly®. In March 2014, I ask my neighbor, David, a retired ophthalmologist, to write a prescription for me for a Cefaly device to test the theory that an electrical distraction may be a migraine cure. I had used a TENS® unit following knee surgery and after manipulation of a frozen shoulder under anesthesia, both painful episodes. A TENS device attaches with sticky electrodes to the skin and diverts me from my acute pain, though relief is fleeting. Imported from Belgium, the Cefaly device cost $349 with three reusable electrodes, and is not covered by medical insurance. Replacement electrodes are $50 for three. It looks like a headband worn over the forehead and attaches to an adhesive backed electrode placed just above my eyebrows in the center of the brow. When the device is turned on, a tingle begins and increases in intensity for a twenty-minute zapping assault. The intensity of the escalating sting may be too much for a patient amid a brainstorm.

On April 17, I begin using Cefaly at bedtime as a migraine preventative. It knocks me out after twenty minutes of bee-stinging and I sleep soundly. At times, I feel relief following a session. Most likely it is a distraction of the nerves, where external prickling masks an internal throb. Other times a migraine blossoms following a session. I have used this device for many months with no noticeable difference in number of headache days and I understand that there is now a Cefaly device indicated for use during acute migraine attacks. But I cannot imagine intentionally stinging my overly sensitive forehead during a brainstorm. However, there are no long-term side effects, and it may be helpful for some migraineurs. April, *nine headache days*.

For twenty-five years I worked for Medtronic, the largest manufacturer of implantable medical devices. The founder of the company, Earl Bakken, developed the first implantable cardiac pacemaker. While touring The Bakken Museum of Medicine and Electricity in Minneapolis, I ask Mr. Bakken which is his most inspirational item in the collection. He points to a book protected under glass. It is a first edition of Mary Shelley's *Frankenstein*. Aha.

My favorite Bakken Museum display is a representation of a primitive treatment for atrial fibrillation. The patient places his feet into a basin of water along with a few slithering electric eels. Current from the eels is conducted through the water, possibly cardioverting an abnormal cardiac rhythm, such as atrial fibrillation. Aha. I have not yet jumped into nearby Lake Michigan during a lightning storm to possibly reset my brain, but sometimes an alternative to modern medicine should be considered.

chapter 17

LET'S GO BLUE

All experience is great providing you live through it. If it kills you, you've gone too far.
—Alice Neel[23]

May 7, at my initial visit to the U of M Adult Neurology and Headache Clinic, I am feeling optimistic about treatment from the "Leaders and Best." The University of Michigan Hospital is ranked in the top ten in the U.S. in certain listings. And so, I drive across the state to submit to Go Blue therapy. Dr. Charleston spends two hours going through my H & P (history and physical). He seems unhurried, though I experienced a long wait as he spent significant time with earlier patients. I feel validated by his focus on my concerns rather than seeing me as the chronic complainer I was to other less patient-centered physicians. Because of his interest and attention to detail, I start to anticipate a cure. I take notes as he tells me to wait twenty-four hours between ingesting any vasoconstrictive drugs to prevent rebounding headaches. "Increase hydration. Dehydration is the #1 cause of headache." Amen. My travel buddy is a refillable, stainless steel insulated water bottle. Doc says "Amerge works faster than Frova® (frovatriptan), but Frova has the longest half-life. Amerge has the second longest half-life of all triptans."

Doc's strategy: "Stay on riboflavin 100mg four times per day. It has been shown to be more effective than placebo. DC butterbur, unless Petadolex®, brand which is PA-free, since that is hepatotoxic." (Butterbur is an herb which naturally contains pyrrolizidine alkaloids, PAs, which can damage the liver, lungs, blood circulation, and possibly cause cancer.) I learn something new here about OTC treatments; some of them are quite toxic just like prescription meds and most lack clinical studies and quality testing.

"Increase CoQ10 to 300mg per day." I nod while I take more notes. Doc continues, "U of M's acute treatment protocol uses a scale of 1-10 for pain. For level 1-3, try non-pharmacological treatment including hydration. For level 4-6, Amerge 2.5mg. You may repeat in two hours, with a maximum use of two days per week. At pain level 7-10: take acetaminophen 1000mg with Phenergan 25mg (an antihistamine which may be synergistic with pain meds, and it diminishes nausea).

If level 7 or above for more than three days, take naproxen 500mg with food. For prophylaxis, switch from magnesium glycinate to magnesium oxide 400mg twice daily as tolerated. Botox may reduce peripheral sensitization. Let's start with 155 units, 31 injections in face, neck, shoulders every 90 days." Sign me up for another round of this pricey toxin.

"DC Midrin. Begin Effexor®." (venlafaxine, a selective serotonin reuptake inhibitor which affects brain chemicals. Indicated use is depression. Off label for migraine prevention.)

"Cefaly. Okay to use at bedtime as a preventative. You may take melatonin 3mg control release tablet two-three hours before bedtime. Return for nerve blocks in 10-12 weeks."

I am not surprised, when Doc suggests a sphenopalatine catheter squirt of lidocaine. Dr. Charleston worked on a clinical study of this treatment with Dr. Strabbing, the ENT I visited in South Haven just prior. I read their clinical study and understand that they would like to see more patients sign up so that the study may gain legs. This is a thirty-minute procedure which requires a driver afterward. Since I do not have a chauffeur to and from Ann Arbor, I decline for now. And I am a bit nervous. The procedure sounds gag-inducing, possibly paralyzing the throat, and dangerous. How could I ask for help if my throat is paralyzed? Doc orders an EKG to check QT segment, a concern with Phenergan (for nausea) use. I am impressed with his caution. My heart checks out a-okay today.

May, *six headache days*. On May 9, I head back to yoga class after a long time away. Namaste. I am blessed with a lovely headache-free vacation for three heavenly weeks until a sneaky sinus infection flares up. Again. I begin a round of Amoxicillin/Clavacillin and a Medrol Dosepak on June 30. Again. June, *five headache days*.

On July 9, I travel from South Bend via Amsterdam to Prague for the first week of my fourth MFA residency. The language is more difficult than any other I have attempted to learn. The taxi driver who picks me up at the airport after my overnight flight tries to engage me with a bit of sign language and pointing, then tunes his radio to a station playing American country music. I cannot tell him that I am no fan of American country music, so I nod and smile as he says, "Kenny Rogers good." My lodging for the first two nights is in the Hotel Century Old Town Prague. I am thrilled to learn that I am sleeping next door to the room where Franz Kafka worked as an insurance underwriter between 1908 and 1922, according to the plaque on the door. One hundred years later I appreciate the Kafkaesque irony of trying to communicate with Czechs I meet with the language barrier and the migraine-erasure of many of my English words. I am reading his autobiographical fiction, *The Castle*. It is a masterpiece of twentieth century existentialism which I find relatable. Immersed in Kafka's dreamscape, I am pushing up against the absurdity of writing each day in my room, next to his, despite the futility of escaping my squeezing skull. Will I survive and achieve meaning or is this pinched brain my own locked-away castle?

As our group travels during the second week by bus to Germany, we watch the 2006 film, *The Lives of Others*. I am astonished by the repression of East Berliners, being spied on by the Stasi as well as their own neighbors and sometimes family members. Our hotel is a few blocks east of Checkpoint Charlie, a well-known heavily guarded border crossing during the cold war. I shudder each time I freely pass through. It is just twenty-five years since this wall fell. And it is a simmering summer to witness Holocaust Memorials. How can I complain of *nine migraine days* in July when I am otherwise free and healthy?

August 8, U of M appointment. Doc says "Cefaly use has not been studied concurrently with Botox injections, so take a break for a few days after the next Botox round. Botox works by paralyzing muscles and Cefaly modulates nerves." Indeed. I receive 31 Botox injections with 155 units into the bilateral corrugator, temporalis, occipitalis, cervical spinal muscles, trapezius, left and right frontalis, and procerus. Discharge instructions: "Taper off Zanaflex (muscle relaxer) over a week. Hydrate well before the next Botox treatment and try Tylenol with 65mg of caffeine (a cup of tea) as needed for headache."

On 8/18 Dr. Strabbing, ENT, orders another CAT scan of my sinuses. Loads of radiation and nothing *treatable* discovered. "Your issues are too close to the brain for safe intervention," says the surgeon. Should I be happy to hear that I am not a surgical candidate?

November 14, Botox 155 units at U of M. January 2015, *twelve headache days*; February, *eight headache days*.

February 13, U of M office visit. February 14, Botox increased to 165 units. It is not possible for me to combine an office visit to discuss treatments along with Botox injections on the same day, so I settle for an overnight stay at Weber's Inn in Ann Arbor with appointments on consecutive days. The Neurology Clinic schedules "procedures" on certain days of the week, so Doc can spend adequate time with each patient. It may work for clinic personnel, but it is a three-hour drive for me to return for multiple appointments. Is this patient-focused quality?

RIP dear mother. Elizabeth Terese Ryan, 1927-2015, escapes her earthly existence, trading pain for peace on March 3, 2015.

March, *four headache days*. April, *fourteen headache days*. May, *eight headache days*. June 15, Botox 155 units.

Flying overnight via Amsterdam to Athens on June 23 for my graduation residency, I pray that summer heat will not broil my brain at 35 degrees latitude. I wear a wide-brimmed hat, sunglasses, and sip water while I take in the Parthenon on the Athenian Acropolis. At Delphi, the womb of the world, I am heat struck and muttering inanities as inscrutable as the ancient oracles, though no one is all that interested in ramblings from a nonfiction MFA candidate. At the navel of civilization on the Isle of Crete, I deliver my graduation lecture, "The Odyssey of Memoir." Thank goodness for air conditioning in hotels. It is as hot, though not as humid as my former home of Louisville in the summer, a sure-migraine trigger. I chill my brain when I can find ice, chug electrolytes out of a thermos, and lie in my air-conditioned single room between classes and tours. Celebrating at the end of the program with three nights on the island of Santorini, I spend two days snorkeling and sailing in the Aegean. The water is bathtub-warm and as clear as Ouzo. The locals say the lack of flora and fauna is due to the nearby simmering volcano and its earlier destructive eruptions. The seabed looks like a rough-surfaced, off-white swimming pool. Though a dark room with an ice pack is calling me, I surrender and embrace this wonder of the world, a once in a lifetime visit to a hot as Hades paradise. Opa!

June, *ten headache days*. July, *nine headache days*. August, *sixteen headache days*. September 14, Botox 155 units. September, *thirteen headache days*.

October, MRI of lower spine following a frightening numbness from hips to toes. Diagnosis: degenerative spine. Yikes, that's old lady back. Treatment: PT exercises for sciatica and numbness. Frequent rounds of steroids prescribed for migraine interruption and sinusitis are not kind to crumbling back bones. October, *sixteen headache days.* November, *two headache days.* December, *two headache days.* December 10, Botox 155 units. January 2016, *five headache days.* February, *two headache days.* March, *eight headache days.*

March 18, Botox increased to 165 units. April, *six headache days.* May, *nine headache days.* June, *seventeen headache days.* July 5, Botox increased to 175 units since I seem to have more frequent headaches in the weeks just before my next round of injections. I experience dizziness after the second occipital injection, a mild premonitory vasovagal response. I recline for the remainder of injections, and I am moved out of the treatment room immediately after receiving my doses to make room for the next patient. Patients are hurried through *à la* assembly line on treatment days in this neurology clinic: no gaps or empty rooms. Just one patient after another. Henry Ford would be impressed with this efficiency. A medical assistant escorts me from the treatment room and seats me at a blood pressure station in the hallway after I tell her I am very dizzy and about to pass out. I say, "Help me to the floor." She ignores my request and continues to try to get a BP reading as I slump. I hear her say I am unresponsive for about 45 seconds, so she calls a code, which means either cardiac arrest or respiratory arrest. No shades of grey here. When I awaken with a crash cart parked near my nose, I am alarmed, and my blood pressure rises to a measurable level. When I worked in the inpatient pharmacy at nearby St. Joseph Hospital, I routinely stocked the crash carts, and I understand the seriousness of calling a code. It may be as likely to kill a patient whose heart has not stopped as to save one whose heart has stopped.

I ask the tech, "Did my heart arrest? Did I stop breathing?"

"No and no."

"You could have killed me with an unnecessary code."

She shrugs and says, "Just following hospital protocol." This is not the first time my cause of death in a hospital could have been caused by "protocol."

This all happened within fifteen minutes of the last Botox injection. Against my protests, I am loaded on a gurney in the Neurology Clinic and carted off to the Emergency Department for observation. Hospital protocol. This is not my idea of how my day would proceed. I was looking forward to lunch at Zingerman's Deli. With my blood pressure rising to readings of 92/53, 102/62, I am still subjected to three hours of waiting in the ER for a physician to release me from the hospital. And I am refused food. My chart is labeled NPO: (*nil per os*) nothing by mouth. Since I missed lunch, I have a crushing brainstorm, and hospital protocol is making it worse by withholding nourishment. I am offered IV fluids. "No thank you. I have had more than enough pokes today. How about a package of crackers, juice, yogurt, tea? My blood sugar is low enough to be the culprit in this migraine."

"Sorry, you are NPO until you see the doctor," says the nurse who checks on me when she is not taking care of a real emergency. The young ER physician, Dr. Mary Eddy, not related to the Christian Science founder, Mary Baker Eddy, checks me out after scanning my EKG, and saying, "Your heart is as healthy as mine." I read her discharge diagnosis, which was the same as mine, "Vasovagal response to 31 injections in the face and neck. Treatment: food and water." I scarf a package of crackers with yogurt and tea before leaving the ER. I nearly melt when I exit the hospital's chilly air conditioning into 92 degree-humid-heat. While searching for my car in the parking garage, I feel shaky, confused, and surprised that after earlier diligent concern for my well-being, I am now wandering alone, dazed in this steamy, fume-filled cavern. Is this patient-focused care? Hospitals are not always the best place to be ill. How about retrieving my car? Next time I will valet park.

July, *five headache days*. August, *eleven headache days*. September, *ten headache days*.

Blue Cross denies payment for two rounds of Botox treatments, saying my "headaches are not chronic." This is an example of what happens when bean counters practice medicine. For eighteen months I try to get this resolved, with a $5000 balance at U of M due to miss-coding I believe. My account is turned over to a collection agency. Blue Cross will not return my calls, and U of M has written me off instead of working it out with Blue Cross. So, I make payments of $50 per month for a very long time. Sometimes I just sing the blues.

October 11: 175 units Botox in 31 sites.

chapter 18

Monoclonal Antibodies

Suffering is the entrance to the person. It is the door to something larger.
—Rumi[24]

I would happily open all my doors and windows
for a cure.
—Susan P. Ryan

An insurance company's refusal to pay for treatment of a common chronic medical condition is contributing to the burden of migraine. Out of frustration and needing more help than a primary care physician can offer, I switch to a less expensive provider than University Hospital, and a closer to home neurologist, Dr. David Erhardt at Hauenstein Neurosciences at St. Mary Hospital, Grand Rapids. Dr E treats me with Botox every 90 days and starts me on the latest FDA approved treatment for migraine prevention: Aimovig® (erebumab-aooe). This is the first drug approved in a class of monoclonal antibodies called CGRP Inhibitors (Calcitonin Gene-Related Peptide Inhibitors). I am his first patient to begin injecting this drug. Doc says, "The sales rep tells me there are *no side effects* and there is a high rate of reduction in frequency and severity of migraine symptoms during clinical studies." My first job after college was as a sales representative for Ayerst, a pharmaceutical company. I understand how reps are taught to minimize negatives and sell the features and benefits of a drug to the prescriber. This makes me skeptical about the claim of *no side effects*. And after several months of injecting myself with this new wonder drug, constipation becomes incapacitating, despite a colonoscopy-type bowel prep regimen each evening. I stop short of dynamite and ask Doc for another option. Lucky for me another CGRP Inhibitor has been FDA approved, Ajovy® (Fremanezumab-vfrm). I stab and inject 4.5cc subcutaneously each month. Depositing nearly a teaspoonful of liquid into the subcutaneous layer of my muscular upper leg is not ideal. I switch my target to belly fat and the swelling from the quail-egg-sized injection resolves a few hours after administration. My co-pay is $720.76.

October, *eight headache days*. November, *ten headache days*. December, *twelve headache days*. January 2017, *eight migraine days*. February, *eight migraine days*. March, *nine headache days*. April, *four headache days*. Yippee! May, *ten headache days*. June, *seventeen headache days*. WHY?

Botox injections on July 11. Will this be my lucky day?

Traveling overnight from Kalamazoo to Edinburgh on

July 12 to join fellow MFA alums and student writers, I begin a Medrol Dosepak to lighten my load of brainstorms on this trip. There is no Scotch whiskey sampling for me, though bites of haggis and the frequent sightings of Scotsmen strutting about in gorgeous kilts are things I cannot enjoy at home. The first day I hike twelve miles solo through botanical gardens, filling my eyes and cameras with lush flora. I savor a meal of local broiled cod with fried capers. After dinner I bypass the lounge where fellow writers are socializing over cocktails and head to my requested "quiet" single room at the end of the hallway. I am tired from my day-long walk and jet-lagged from overnight travel and hope to enjoy a headache-free trip. Sheer curtains filter a fresh breeze while the sun barely sets at latitude 55.57 degrees. Birds chatter all night in the midsummer courtyard, making up for their silence in dark winter, and I join in their sleeplessness. In addition to a scrambled circadian rhythm from time-zone travel, an energizing steroid burst, and a not quite dark night keep me awake. After counting Scottish sheep, and reading all the books in my room, I think about the movie *Insomnia*, a thriller set in an Alaskan summer, starring Robin Williams, Hilary Swank, and Al Pacino. The inability to sleep due to the midnight sun is mind-threatening for the visiting investigator from Los Angeles. But I have decided that insomnia due to so much daylight is just part of my adventure.

On Saturday I hike with the alumni group "The Mile" to Holyrood. Alas, the queen is not available for tea today. The next day we hike up Arthur's Seat for a panoramic view of city and sea. Thrilled to be an alumnus, I take in all offered tours instead of sitting each day in classes in an unexplored country. Our Scottish guide John prances up the mountain in kilt and boots, fleece jacket and scarf. In his thick Scots accent, he warns of the "kelpies, who can take on the form of anything, horses perhaps. They take children to the sea and drown them and eat them." Oh, my! He explains another bit of lore concerning "a beautiful naked woman by the water's edge. When a man tries to touch her, he is dragged away to the river and drowned." John's tales are tall and thirst-provoking. I swill electrolytes and hike 96 stories according to my iPhone app. We straddle the earth's edge, where two tectonic plates merged eons ago and hop like kangaroos from rock to rock. Attempting to unfurl a Scottish flag for a photo op, our team is nearly blown off the peak.

The following day the entire group of students, alums, and faculty travel in two buses across the narrow country, landing in Glasgow about fifty miles away. My highlight is hiking through fragrant gardens surrounding Culzean Castle, overlooking the Firth of Clyde. In 1945 the Marquess of Ailzan presented the castle and its surrounding gardens to the National Trust for Scotland, and he requested that a portion of the castle be offered to General Eisenhower in gratitude from the Scottish people for leading the Allied Forces during WWII. We are told that Eisenhower enjoyed his stays here, though he returned this "gift" after the war. On my next visit to Scotland, I hope to visit the Hebrides archipelago and play a round of golf at St. Andrews. On this trip my record is .500 against migraine with steroids batting clean-up. It is as disappointing as playing bogey golf for a pro, though it is not so bad for me with my lower expectation.

July, *eleven headache days*. August, *ten headache days*. September, *twelve headache days*. October, *eleven headache days*. November, *ten headache days.* December, *nine headache days.* January 2018, *sixteen headache days.*

I visit with Dr. Ehrhardt for Botox injections and follow-up on January 18. Doc recommends: "Use Relpax® (eletriptan) with Compazine® (prochlorperazine), an anti-nausea medication for migraine. Always take two drugs together to abort an attack. And take the meds earlier rather than letting the migraine take control." Sure. But I like to wish the rascals away, telling myself that *it is just a headache* when the initial pangs surface. I often hold off on taking abortive meds, trying to conserve my twice weekly allowed triptan doses, though I often fail to guess right and fall into an unresponsive migraine that lingers for two or three days. It is difficult for me to know when symptoms foretell a real brainstorm, but most of the time they unfortunately do.

February, *thirteen headache days.* March, *five headache days.* April, *eleven headache days.* Botox injections on April 25. May, *six headache days.* June, *nine headache days.* July, *fifteen headache days.* August, *eight headache days.* September, *nine headache days.* October, *ten headache days.* Botox injections on October 26 with a Toradol injection for a migraine underway during my office visit with the neurologist. November, *9 headache days.* December, *9 headache days.*

On December 9, I switch to a second CGRP inhibitor, Ajovy® (fremanezumab-vfrm), and have *9 consecutive days free of headache.* Cure or coincidence? January 2019, *seven headache days.* On January 25, Botox injections with my latest neurologist Dr. Audrey Sanders. Dr. Ehrhardt moved away from this clinic. I have *eleven consecutive headache-free days.* Ole. February, *seven headache days.* March, *eight headache days.* April, *five headache days.*

Sarah Dykema N.P. administers Botox on 4/25 in Grand Haven, closer to home. She also works for the Hauenstein Neurosciences Center. I have not switched providers. May, *three headache days* and I move from my South Haven home where ubiquitous short-term vacation rentals with requisite backyard bonfires choke out the neighbors on most summer nights. A smoky haze hangs over the land as I paddle my kayak offshore and breathe more easily away from the smoke. Every spring, summer, and fall my neighborhood becomes party-central for vacationers. Residential zoning is not enforced by the City of South Haven and commercial enterprises have taken over most blocks. Fighting city hall for several years, I realize that this is not how I want to spend my retirement. So, I move. Again. My new residence is in West Olive, forty-five miles north, with neighborhood stairs down a dune to Lake Michigan, and adjacent to a county park with miles of hiking trails. I choose this location because my new subdivision does not allow short-term rentals. This rule has already been tested by a lawsuit, so I hope and pray that this will be my permanent perch. May this blessing extinguish my brainstorms.

On June 11, I travel to Maine for the weekend to attend the wedding of Elizabeth and Abe. Elizabeth is the daughter of my Medtronic friend Karen. I have one or two glasses of wine and gallons of water during the entire weekend of celebration. I am a wet blanket, placing my hand over my glass whenever the server offers a pour. Everyone around me is festive while I slip on my well-practiced salesperson smile, trying to cover up my affliction. Yes, I have a migraine during much of the visit.

The Spalding MFA program is generous in inviting alumni back for courses in Louisville and travel abroad. I travel to Santiago, Chile July 7 to 19 with fellow writers. It is winter in the Southern Hemisphere, and the climate suits my brain better than past summer writing residencies in Europe. Not so long ago I was an avid skier with a fantasy of schussing down South America's slopes during summer, but I am satisfied with this literary trip and a bit of hiking. My knees have schussed over too many miles of rugged terrain, so I have relegated my favorite sport to my dreams. I enjoy a couple of Pisco Sours during the twelve-day trip and feel no ill effect. But the Chilean wines are not so kind. Though I may be a bit dehydrated since we are hiking at higher altitudes in the Andes while visiting slope side vineyards and my water bottle seems to be empty whenever I am miles from a refillable source. I lug home a bottle of Pisco and concoct a batch of Pisco Sours to celebrate summer with my sisters on my Michigan patio. This South American brandy concoction tastes like a Margarita without the head-slamming proclivity of tequila. I limit myself to a rare single alcoholic drink and sometimes escape without a migraine. Sometimes.

I undergo allergy skin testing on July 31 with dozens of itchy pokes so the allergist can update my biweekly serum. I read that researchers suggest that migraine may be an autoimmune-type disorder. Could something like an allergy shot be in the future arsenal for migraineurs?

May, *three headache days*. June, *eleven headache days*. July, *five headache days*. August 1, Botox injections. August, *seven headache days*. September, *six headache days*. October, *three headache days*. November 7, Botox injections. November, *ten headache days*. December, *five headache days*.

My insurance provider for Part D Medicare (prescription drug coverage) is switched without my input. I am no longer eligible to receive Ajovy, even though it seems to be reducing the frequency and severity of my headaches. This drug is now considered "non-formulary." I am instructed by the insurer to go back on Aimovig despite its life-threatening severe constipation complication. No way. The insurer must have negotiated a darn good deal on this drug, since other patients have complained of this intolerable side effect and demand for the drug is diminishing. I call Shelly R.N. at the neurology office, and she intervenes. I am switched to a third CGRP inhibitor, Emgality® (galcanezamab), recently FDA approved. WellCare allows it for three months only. Do they expect a cure for my chronic condition in 90 days? Sounds perfect. The copay is $362, and I am diverted to another pharmacy twelve miles from home. How inconvenient for a patient who should not drive during dizzy brainstorms and this drug cannot be mailed since it must be kept refrigerated. I understand that insurance companies have a profit motive, but what about their customers, patients who are suffering and paying monthly premiums? Third party non-medically trained individuals are playing doctor, but their primary concern is compensation. Let us remove this unnecessary layer of thieves. Whenever I experience an improvement in the quality of my life, insurance companies intervene and swap therapies on me. I am not a generic person. I do not need your choice of generic drug. And why are so many of the generic drugs you foist on us made in China and India? I have experienced quality issues with several of these imports which I will cover in a later chapter.

If consumers directly pay physicians, hospitals, and pharmacies, we could eliminate the bulging-pocketed middlemen, saving money and aggravation. I am not in favor of Medicare for all since the resulting rationing of healthcare will override any benefit of cost savings like it has in European and Canadian healthcare systems. During my career in the medical device industry, I saw firsthand how patients waited on queue until they were no longer candidates for heart valve replacements in these countries. They had become too ill, too old, or died while awaiting their procedure. But enough grousing about something I cannot correct. Perhaps it is time for an off-road adventure.

chapter 19

THE CANNABIS CURE

Organic chemistry is the chemistry of carbon compounds. Biochemistry is the study of carbon compounds that crawl.
—Mike Adams[25]

To acquire medical marijuana in the Great Lakes State (this is a year or so before recreational pot shops sprout like Starbucks™ every six blocks), one must obtain a Michigan Medical Marihuana Card. The State of Michigan uses the archaic spelling in legal documents, with "h" in place of the more common "j." The State Licensing site claims that this spelling is derived from the Marihuana Tax Act of 1937. While the botanical name cannabis was the nomenclature of physicians and pharmacists of that time, the federal government decided to relabel marijuana, derived from the Spanish *mariguana,* and further anglicized it to marihuana to accommodate the American tongue. The foreign sounding slang may have been an effort to denigrate centuries of cannabis use as a medically accepted treatment.

My primary care provider is sympathetic to my research, understanding that I have run out of options to treat my chronic migraine. But since she works for a hospital corporation which frowns on this quasi-legal alternative treatment, she is unable to sign my application form for a MMM License. This hospital organization permits patients almost any prescription to ameliorate pain, but not Schedule I demon weed. For Schedule II Demerol®, Fioricet, Morphine, Percocet®, or Oxycontin®, just sign here. Opioids are us.

My physician listens to my litany of side effects from meds that give no abatement and offers what she can. "The next time you have a bad migraine, come by the office for an injection of ketorolac." This butt-burning intramuscular anti-inflammatory injection takes the edge off, but it does not conquer my head pain. I have received shots of ketorolac during doctor visits that coincided with a migraine, and I have injected myself a dozen times in the thigh since I am not dexterous enough to inject my own gluteus maximus. I have found this pain in the ass to be merely a short-term distraction for migraine. She continues. "Just ask the office to squeeze you in and you shouldn't have to wait much more than an hour."

I know that I am unlikely to choose this option, since even the short drive to her office and sitting for an hour or more in a waiting room are not compatible with dizziness, nausea, severe headache, and vomiting. Doc emails a prescription to the local

Walgreen for another Medrol Dosepak, a steroid which may break up a weeks-long migraine, though it is not a drug to be used frequently, since one of its side effects is bone-thinning, a definite no-no with my already thin bones. Though Doc supports my quest for medical marihuana, she cannot give me advice since her prescription-writing hands are shackled by her employer. She says *sotto voce*, "Why don't you travel to Colorado or California, where medical marihuana has been available for several years. There will be more medical practitioners to advise you. But of course, you'll not be able to leave Colorado or California with cannabis. You'll need to acquire your stash in Michigan."

I search online and locate a clinic about an hour drive from my home where a licensed physician can authorize me to apply for a Michigan Medical Marihuana Patient Card. His specialty is pot procurement. Office hours begin after 5 pm and next day appointments are available for a $95 fee. No insurance accepted.

The next evening as I pull into the parking lot of the so-called Wellness Clinic, I assess the run-down strip mall, and its questionable enterprises: "Lose Weight Fast," "Tattoos While You Wait," "Pay Day Loans," and "Cash for Plasma." These businesses invoke a sense of urgency, but is not my search for a migraine cure also urgent? I reflect on approaching similar seedy looking offices during my first job after college when I detailed pharmaceuticals in Detroit for a Fortune 500 company. I developed survival instincts on the job which may have protected me from harm during thirty years of traveling solo in iffy areas. Whenever bad vibes tingled through my core, I remained in the car and missed out on danger or opportunities. But if the sun dazzled and I felt adventurous, I would grab my detail bag and buzz at locked doors for admittance.

The short wavelengths of February twilight are fading in West Michigan and Arctic air pinches my nose as I leave the warmth of my car. Though I park near the door, I consider backing into the parking space for a speedier departure. I am not paranoid, just practical. Prior experience lends caution to my decisions. As I open the door to the office, my glasses fog with condensation from the temperature differential. I take them off and wait for them to clear so I can navigate through the dim room. It is a dark cave, perfect for migraineurs or bats. Squinting, I spy three or four male patients seated in folding chairs, with the light of smart phones illuminating their youthful faces. They all appear young enough to be my grandsons. Consciously or not, we all evaluate people at first glance. Natural selection has taught us to categorize others, to size them up. Will fight or flight be necessary in this encounter? Can I remain calm, or should I prepare for a confrontation? As a seasoned sales professional, ever reading others, I wonder why these young men are visiting such a clinic. Perhaps they are fellow migraineurs. We do not look ill to the casual observer. But the young men in this waiting room do not fit the typically female migraine profile. Must be another malady. *Do not judge them.* But I smile while I muse about their thoughts of me visiting this place, though they probably do not even see me, an older woman, no one of interest. I am invisible.

After a brief wait, a disheveled doctor reeking of cigarette smoke escorts me into his office and scans my completed form. He looks worn out, unkempt in a wrinkled shirt, under a dingy lab coat, no tie, un-doctorly, and again my mind categorizes him in this makeshift office.

He asks, "What brings you here today?"

"Chronic migraine, about fifteen days each month. Standard treatments do not help, and the side effects are worse than the headache."

"Have you ever tried cannabis for migraine?"

"No, but I am at the end of my rope."

"And how long have you experienced migraine?"

"Since I was twelve."

"Why did you wait so long?"

"Lack of clear dosage information, questionable strength of active ingredients, purity, basically safety and efficacy. There is also the Schedule I concern: fear of the Feds and possibly losing my drive and creativity, fuzzy cognition, and deleterious effects on my lungs."

Doc does not say a word, so I continue. "Can you give me advice on routes of administration, optimal ratio of CBD/THC for migraine prevention, best strains for my brain, and also treatment for acute headache?"

"I'm not familiar with treatments," he says. But I doubt it. He looks like someone who has experienced more than a few mind-altering intoxicants. A tremor ripples over his hands as he signs my form. "Chronic pain is your diagnosis." Indeed. Doc appears to be near my age, close to retirement, and not a stranger to hard living. As he escorts me to the door, he asks, "What's with the briefcase?"

"Medical records. The web site said to bring documentation of medical need."

Doc barks a smoker's laugh. He has not examined me in any way. No blood pressure cuff, no stethoscope, no peering into my eyes or ears. He never touches me. Not even a handshake. He just fills out the form and signs it. I read that only 6 percent of all cannabis consumed or smoked in the U.S. is for medicinal purposes. I am a hopeful outlier.

However, I must say something in defense of the good doctor who signs my MMML form and sends me on my way with "Good luck." By federal law, physicians are not permitted to give advice on how to use a Schedule I drug such as heroin, marihuana, peyote, LSD, or Ecstasy. They are all considered by the DEA to have *"no currently accepted medical use and a high potential for abuse."* However, cocaine, fentanyl, and oxycontin are all Schedule II, so, guidance on these drugs is allowable. Medical marihuana patients are relegated to online sources for treatment tips and in print from *High Times*, *Weed World*, and *Cannabis Now* magazines, which I recently picked up at Barnes and Noble™ along with boxes of Christmas cards. The clerk at the register gave me a strange look. "Research," I said to her with a straight face and "Merry Christmas." There is a dearth of clinical studies compared to plentiful data on Schedule II-V and non-scheduled drugs. Pharmacists cannot dispense weed, nor can they recommend dosage, appropriate plant genus, and monitor drug-drug interactions. Purity is not guaranteed and contamination by pesticide and fungicide residues is probable. Indoor growing increases the likelihood of moldy weed, a serious health hazard for anyone, and especially someone with a compromised immune system. Extractions are often obtained via butane and other cheap solvents, which an informed consumer would not willingly ingest. Organic weed? It is unlikely to meet standards set by the USDA for agricultural products, since the government does not yet inspect cannabis growers. It is after all, still federally illegal. Buyer beware.

As someone who spent four years in pharmacy school, worked in the healthcare industry for over thirty years, and rarely consumes alcohol, it is surely desperation that drives me to acquire a license to score dope for my chronic condition. Headaches have taken over my life for too many years. And now that I am retired, it is time to find a cure. A long, strange journey leads me to the doorstep of the nearest medical marihuana dispensary late on a Saturday afternoon, a few hours after the mailman delivers my license to buy, my ticket to ride. During the fifty-mile drive, I laugh out loud, wondering what my family would say if they were along for this ride. The parking lot is packed, and the neighborhood is seedy. Pun intended. I am afraid to leave my well-groomed standard poodle in the minivan at the lone parking space I find at the rear of the business, so I park illegally in front of Sid's Smoke Shop next door. A sign says "Customer Parking Only. Violators Towed." But with cinched blinds on the windows, the business appears closed, so I park illegally. I am living a bit dangerously today.

The Buddery building is painted a faded shade of Crayola™ blue both inside and out and the plate glass windows beg for a quart of Windex™. A bubbly young woman greets me in a musical voice at the check-in desk. She seems overjoyed to be working here. Her employer must offer great benefits.

"Welcome to your first visit to the Buddery. I'm making up a packet just for you, with info about special events and discounts (green stamps, coupons, frequent flyer points). May I have your Michigan Driver's License and your Michigan Medical Marihuana License? I'll make a copy and get them right back to you." Do these two permits even belong in the same wallet?

After a short wait, I am escorted behind a locked door into the inner sanctum, which reeks of the wares. I sneeze and my eyes dart to the rear of the building as I search for an exit—just in case. The scout's motto of "Be Prepared" trips through my head as I am directed to station #3.

"Susan, I'm Dave, your personal budtender. I hope you're carrying enough cash. The ATM in the lobby is empty and we don't take credit cards. It's always empty on Saturdays 'cause people are stocking up for the weekend, ya' know." I nod. I feel as if I am visiting a movie set, though the skunk aroma is all too real. Looking into Dave's red, white, and blue eyes, I realize that he is rather stoned. An occupational hazard. He mentions that his father is coming to visit this evening from across the state. Why is he bringing up his father? He must be trying to relate to me. He's using a Sales 101 strategy. I am feeling a bit maternal toward this young man while I wonder what Dave's Dad thinks of his son's budtending. Since the Buddery is just outside of a college town, I wonder if Dave dropped out of school for this career opportunity. I do not ask but redirect my attention to the shopping experience.

"Let's take a quick tour." He shows me infused honey "for your tea," gummy bears, hard candies, capsules, oils, extractions, creams, roll-ons, and jars and jars of lovely flowers, glowing with their potential magic. This scene reminds me of a fabulous and tempting candy shop from my childhood. Dave interrupts my reverie.

"So, what are you looking to treat?"

"Chronic migraine."

"Cool. I get headaches too. These flowers—Girl Scout Cookies is the variety—give me relief in minutes. Roll up a nice doobie, take a few hits, and wait for the effect before continuing. We have rolling papers for joints or pre-rolled blunts in cigar paper made from tobacco leaves. And we have pipes too, regular and water pipes."

"But I don't want to damage my lungs. I have allergies and asthma."

"Cool. Yeah, weed makes me sneeze a lot, but it really helps with my ADD. It's a trade-off." He directs me to the next jar of flowers and invites me to take a whiff as he lifts the lid. "If you need to super focus, I recommend these Purple Kush flowers."

Another sneeze after sniffing the Kush. "I'll keep that in mind for my next visit, but let's start with something I don't need to smoke."

"For the health-conscious consumer, we recommend a vaporizer, which heats herbs to a temperature high enough to extract THC, CBD, and other beneficial cannabinoids, but these temps are too low for the potentially harmful toxins that are released during combustion. Essentially, vaporization minimizes the health risks associated with smoking. And it reduces odor. It's more discreet for the discriminating consumer."

I try not to laugh at Dave's choice of phrases: minimizing health risks, discriminating and health-conscious consumer. I have been in few places less discriminating than this backroom. And health risks? Ha. Who knows? Spin the roulette wheel. But his spiel does remind me of my early days detailing pharmaceuticals, where we minimized side effects and focused on features and benefits to make a sale. This Buddery is big business in dirty blue jeans. And just like Big Pharma, they too rely on Marketing 101 techniques.

"Thanks for the info but I really don't want to inhale anything."

"Cool, ma'am. Tinctures are liquid cannabis extract, which will give you dosage control and fast-acting effects without the health risks associated with smoking. Just 3-4 drops under the tongue. This will be instantly absorbed, giving you rapid relief. No pass through the liver."

"Yeah, I remember about routes of administration and first pass effect from pharmacy school, but I don't want to be buzzed, just relieved of migraine."

"Sure. You'll want a higher ratio of CBD to THC since CBD is anti-inflammatory and THC is the psychoactive portion of cannabis."

"Okay. Let's see a CBD tincture."

"Not in stock today."

"Right."

"Maybe an ingestible oil, a happy medium between edibles and concentrates. RS Oil originated in 2003 when Rick Simpson concocted concentrated extracts to cure his skin cancer."

"Is it THC-free?"

"Nope."

"Let's move on then."

"You could apply a topical to your temples or wherever the pain is. Since it treats locally, the THC won't bother your mind."

This phrase rings in my head like a Bob Dylan lyric but I cannot place it. *Won't bother your mind.*

"Yes. I'll try a jar of the orange-scented Michigan Magic Rub."

"Great stuff. I use it all the time for injuries. My left ankle, knee, and back were pretty messed up last week, but it's really helping."

"Did you lose a fight with your girlfriend?"

"No, I fell down the stairs. I'm clumsy. I fall a lot."

"Sorry to hear that."

"No worries."

"And a bottle of CBD 10mg capsules for prevention, please. I read that CBD binds to endocannabinoid receptors."

[The EC system was discovered in 1992 by Raphael Mechoulam in Israel who said, "I believe cannabinoids represent a medical treasure waiting to be discovered." And decades later we are still driving blind with this entire class of psychoactive substances because they cannot be patented.]

"Excellent choice. And you should take some candy for when the pain hits. You'll be happy to have it on hand."

"CBD only, please."

"Yes, ma'am."

"This package of Sweet Stone Watermelon candies says 'CBD infused' on the front label, and on the reverse, it says it contains 100mg THC for ten pieces. So which label is correct?"

"The front label is right; it's only CBD, no THC."

Clearly the FDA has not edited the labels nor assayed the content. I wonder what the little gems really contain besides loads of sugar. Are these Jolly Rancher™ knockoffs for the stoner set or children?

"Dave, what type of extraction process is used on your wares? Carbon dioxide, ethanol, or hydrocarbon solvent?"

"Wow. That's a good question. Probably butane."

So probably lighter fluid will be absorbed into a patient's lungs while vaping. What an interesting process for a so-called medical treatment for the not so discriminating consumer. Butane is designated as GRAS, generally recognized as safe by the FDA, though Canada and some U.S. counties have enacted or are considering bans on hydrocarbon extractions. I peel off a wad of bills, and Dave hands me a triple-stapled bag emblazoned with the warning: "Do not open until you reach your final destination." Or cruising altitude. I stuff the goods into my cross-body purse, exit through the security door, and dart through the waiting room, which is crowded with men. The room reeks of smoke and skunk and the rumpled characters remind me of patients who visited the basement pharmacy of St. Joseph Mercy Hospital in the 1970s, where I worked as a pharmacy intern. I would keep one finger on the emergency call button while I waited on recovering junkies. They showed up in the outpatient pharmacy to down their doses of Methadone in Tang™ (orange juice of the astronauts) to prevent recidivism. If the Buddery waiting room fellows tackle me and grab my goody bag, they will be terribly disappointed. They may laugh at me: the old lady is afraid of the buzz. I double-click the locks of my Honda Odyssey and speed off into a darkening March gloom, seeking my final destination. I have scored, but only time will tell if it was worth the effort.

Searching for more in-depth guidance in this nouveau migraine treatment, I take a road trip across the state to Ann Arbor for an appointment with a Cannabis Counselor/Dosage

Specialist. The counselor's business card says she has an M.A. degree. When I ask questions about bioavailability, first pass effect, and solvents used in the vaping process, I realize that she has not taken courses in pharmacology, though perhaps the social sciences. She is very kind and suggests I try vaping for "health benefits. It's easier on your lungs than smoking." I am not so keen on inhaling heated butane vapor, but I watch as she demonstrates vaping CBD, and I try to imagine myself doing so while battling a brainstorm.

"You can apply the $125 office visit fee toward purchase of cannabis products." My cannabis counselor prescribes: "Vaporize with 1:1 Master Kush Indica: Take 2-4 puffs when symptoms start. Wait 5-10 minutes. If the desired effect is not reached, inhale another 2-4 puffs. Repeat as needed, typically in 2-4 hours." The device does not work at home when I try it during a raging brainstorm. "For severe headaches," she prescribes "Indica THC 500mg/jar in peanut butter. It's quite potent, so take one-eighth teaspoonful, which is approximately 5mg on a cracker and wait for thirty minutes to see how you feel before ingesting more."

I pick up "high quality CBD" 10mg capsules as prophylactic treatment and stay on this regimen three times daily for several months. I am advised to use "indica varieties of cannabis and perhaps move to a hybrid with sativa down the road." To abort an incoming migraine, I am sold a glycerin tincture with a high concentration of THC to drop under the tongue for quick absorption. I grab Onya Balm THC, in a twist up container like a deodorant stick, to apply topically to my temples during migraine. I find it eases lower back pain and minimizes the throb of a torn medial collateral ligament in my left knee. This topical seems to me the most effective and predictable mode of administration, and without side effects, though a lingering aroma of skunk settles into my sheets. I sleep better after using the balm on my low back to relieve sciatica.

However, the peanut butter THC is another story. Though taking CBD three times per day for several weeks as a preventative, I continue to endure frequent, intense headaches. One evening while trapped in the embrace of a mother migraine, I pull out the jar of magic peanut butter, dose one-eighth of a teaspoon onto a Triscuit® and wash it down with a glass of water. I wait in bed for the drug to kick in. My heart begins to pound. I feel flushed and overheated. Blood rushes audibly behind my eardrums. I breathe rapidly and experience severe dizziness and nausea. The headache escalates and the side effects continue for several hours. As I too well know, sometimes a treatment is worse than the malady. I am not convinced that oral or inhaled cannabis is safe and effective for me.

Since the highly recommended vape-pen is nonfunctional, I visit another cannabis emporium closer to home and I am offered the "Senior Discount" for purchase of the replacement pen. They hand me a "Free Pre-Roll." Sounds like sushi.

I ask, "What's in it?"

"Whatever we were rolling at the time." *Whatever*. This is not like anything taught in pharmacy school.

"So, what is the dosage?"

They laugh at my naivete, or is it their ignorance? Unconcern? There is no answer as my question hangs in the skunky air. This location offers cannabis seedlings for purchase, with spindly plants placed enticingly at the cash counter, reminding me of houseplants and tired bouquets at the Aldi™ checkout.

Each of the three procurement places I visit has a different vibe and clientele. The Kzoo pot place felt like a head shop from the 70s where one could buy incense to mask cannabis aroma in the dorm. The Ann Arbor emporium was run by women who seemed more caring, attempting to cater to legitimate health issues. The third shop was strictly in it for the buzz.

I cannot recommend nor deny that cannabis may help an individual migraineur, but I do not desire to be daily stoned. I am painfully out of my mind many days each month with migraine, and do not want to waste any more of my conscious time being mentally compromised. However, I keep a topical in my medicine cabinet for occasional relief and I seem to sleep better after applying the balm to my temples, or whatever body part complains the loudest. Cannabis modulates patients' perception of their pain, much like opiates. It does not cancel pain, or cure disease. It works on the central and peripheral nervous system, with analgesic properties, a slowing of dopamine neuro transmission, and it *decreases immune function!* No thank you.

The gold standard of the prospective randomized trial is not available for cannabis treatments. Quality control is inadequate, dosage standards are non-existent, and reported results are generalized anecdotal. This is not a scientific method of reporting data. The question to ask oneself is, do the benefits outweigh the risks? There are documented side effects of heart and lung damage in addition to the decrease in immune function. Recent MRI studies suggest shrinkage of white matter in the brain. Cannabis is not an innocuous drug. It is an under the counter remedy and I would say, buyer beware until we have prospective randomized studies, reliable quality control, and established safety and efficacy for patients.

chapter 20

There Must Be Fifty Ways to Leave Your Migraine

Glory lies in the attempt to reach one's goal and not in reaching it.
—Mahatma Gandhi[26]

A new study reported in *Neurology, Psychiatry and Brain Research*, February 2019, proclaims "Rethinking of the Concepts: Migraine is an Autoimmune Disease." Sure. It could be the next pathophysiology path to pursue. And perhaps migraine will someday be treated like allergies with immunotherapy. Maybe the allergist will include it with my bi-monthly pollen and dust mite desensitization injection. I await the next healing option from modern medicine.

I am currently injecting a new drug every thirty days, Emgality® (galcanezumab-gnlm), a calcitonin-gene related peptide antagonist. This is the third monoclonal antibody I try. It is basically a protein collection, which works on the lining of the brain. According to the manufacturer, Eli Lilly, "Emgality is a *humanized* monoclonal antibody that binds to calcitonin-gene-related peptide (CGRP) and blocks its binding to the receptor." Like insulin, this injection is subcutaneous, and easy to administer. Since I began injecting this "humanized" treatment, I find that my pain level is reduced from the level I endured before using this drug, but the headache frequency has not decreased. I still live with suboptimal symptoms of diminished mental acuity and aphasia, with my head feeling like a soccer ball oozing air after a hard-fought high school game. I endure hangover, complete with nausea, dizziness, fuzzy cognition, and amnesia. I feel depleted. Did I enjoy my last 12 hours by partying? Nope. Do I deserve this serving of humble pie? No alcohol was served, just a changing weather pattern, a low pressure rolling in off Lake Michigan and blowing out all my windows. Again. So, does this expensive new drug work? I believe the pain volume may be reduced by a few decibels and I am afraid to discontinue treatment for fear that the pain will return to its prior intensity. Same with the Botox injections I endure every 90 days—less severe pain but frequent migraine persists.

Immediately after receiving 30+ Botox pokes, a migraine moves in. I cancel plans for the day or three and sofa surf wearing sunglasses. After five to seven days, the toxin's effect has reached its apogee, and a welcome numbness reduces the ability of my nerve endings to incite terror. I have dull headaches, rather than head-banging ones. The pain level is dialed down, giving me some relief, but I still experience cognitive fuzziness, dizziness, and nausea for an average of ten to twelve days per month. It is not a cure for me, but it makes my life incrementally better for about two and a half months. Then I wait through two weeks of intense brainstorms in between treatments since medical insurance companies dictate my pain schedule and sometimes refuse to pay. The official denial letter says, "not medically necessary." Probably issued by a bean-counter without a smidgen of medical knowledge, deciding that Botox injections are for cosmetic reasons. I try to reason with these regulators when I can get one on the phone, explaining my chronic pain and the relief they are denying. But it is nearly impossible to get an actual denier on the phone. Must be too busy as judge and jury. No cross examination. I have learned that prior authorization should be requested by the medical provider to the insurance provider and the treatment itself should be specifically coded "for treatment of chronic migraine," which is an approved indication with most insurance policies. I believe that the insurers make it difficult for patients to receive benefits, hoping that they will give up and pay out of pocket for their treatments, which I sometimes do. The more money they hold onto from patients' monthly premium payments, the bigger their bonuses. And though the insurance companies receive a discount off the list price, there is no discount for the patient paying cash.

Euphoria: On days without brainstorm I tend to forget the brutality of migraine. I cherish my pain-free moments, but I am afraid to make long-term plans. My new normal is several days per week with migraine, depending on weather patterns. Just as I cannot hold off the weather, I cannot postpone the next migraine. Just live through it is my mantra.

Dr. Peter Goadsby of the American Headache Society says

"Migraine is an inherited episodic brain disease. It doesn't shorten life: it ruins it. It affects our most productive people in their most productive years." I appreciate Dr. Goadsby's empathy.

As an eternal optimist, I am not a quitter. I am a problem-solver, not a victim. I worked thirty years in medical sales and have always looked forward to my next opportunity. "No" was a challenge that I accepted. And I still do battle each day in my quest for better health and fewer migraine days. I search for rainbows after the storm has thrashed me and tossed my shipwrecked brain upon the beach. I sip electrolyte solutions with a potassium/sodium ratio of 2:1. No side effects and it may perk me up. Lord knows I can use an infinite amount of hydration after hourly urination while my brain attempts to offload swelling during each siege.

If my environment is noisy, I wear chilled earplugs that I store in the refrigerator. My sensitive eyes hide behind sunglasses on sunny and cloudy days and sometimes indoors. If you cannot feel good, you can at least give the appearance of being cool. If overhead lights are the wrong color temperature, flickering, or otherwise irritating, replace them. Incremental steps add up to a more soothing environment for a sensitive brain.

Cool or warm packs on the head and neck are soothing. I usually prefer ice on my head and warmth on tight neck muscles.

Caffeine: To some migraine specialists it is taboo. But I believe neurologist Dr. Ehrhardt who recommends the same (reasonable) amount each day at the same time. I begin my day with one cup of pour over coffee with breakfast and enjoy a second cup with lunch. My sometimes third cup may be Irish or green tea, but always before 3pm. Sleep is my fickle BFF and requires respect.

Supplements I have tried: At the farmer's market last weekend, I hand over too much cash to the vendor for my fresh greens and he hands me back a few crumpled bills. I mumble, "Thanks. I have a migraine, and my brain is not firing on all cylinders."

Farmer Steve says, "I have just the cure for you." He pours a wee measure of *St. Steve's Wild Bergamot Cordial* into a dose cup, adds hot water from a thermos, and hands it to me. I down it and purchase a bottle of his *Farm-Crafted St. Steve* potion. I admire his marketing acumen.

A few minutes later I turn to my niece nurse Colleen, and mumble, "I am a bit dizzy. Just letting you know in case I head toward the pavement." The morning is heating up on this last Saturday of July and I may be in the early stages of either heatstroke or a cure. I do feel better after cooling off in the airconditioned climate of my Honda Odyssey. And I will test this remedy again. Small improvements are most welcome from any source.

Butterbur has had no effect for me after two years.

I keep a stash of ginger chews in my car, purse, desk, or pocket for whenever the first inkling of nausea occurs. They are a bit helpful and a tasty distraction.

Peppermint is also useful during episodes of pain and nausea. I drink peppermint tea and have consumed peppermint capsules. Applying topical peppermint to the temples soothes the beast, and I have a jar of peppermint cream on my nightstand for nocturnal brainstorms. I try to keep the balm from migrating into my eyes during sleep. Advocates of aroma therapy suggest that peppermint makes one less aware of pain and lavender may lower anxiety if applied to wrists and temples during migraine attacks.

Aveda makes a lipstick-sized peppermint oil roll-on that I carry in my purse.

Feverfew is an herb with no apparent influence on me other than a bit of sneezing. I took it for two years.

Co-Q-10: I take 300mg per day. It is an antioxidant produced by the body, with claims to lower cholesterol, reduce muscle pain, and migraine, and helps to generate energy in cells. I do not know if these claims are true, but since my cholesterol could be lower, I am staying the course. And since production of this nutrient decreases with age, I spend money on this supplement for its supposed energy boost. It is not expensive at Costco.

Magnesium: This mineral is believed to be deficient in migraineurs. It eases vasoconstriction and other headache inducing effects. There are many different magnesium compounds, each with varying properties of absorption. I prefer oral magnesium glycinate. When you find one that your gut tolerates, dosing of once, twice, or three times per day may be beneficial. Soaking in an Epsom salt bath, which is magnesium sulfate, is one of my bedtime treats. It may enhance sleep by allowing the skin to absorb this essential nutrient without overloading a sensitive tummy.

Vitamin B-2, aka Riboflavin, is a water-soluble vitamin, thought to lessen inflammation in the brain. I take 100mg with each meal and at bedtime. It is well tolerated, inexpensive, and I have not experienced any side effects other than bright yellow urine.

Vitamin D deficiency is linked to inflammation in the brain. Living in a northern climate, and wearing sunscreen in summer, I may be deficient if I do not consume additional D-3. Since this vitamin is not water soluble, the dosage should be kept in the range of 1000-5000IU per day. I am currently taking 5000IU each morning. Your physician can order a level of this vitamin with your next blood panel.

Melatonin is a hormone produced in the pineal gland of the brain, responsible for setting one's sleep clock. Some studies show that low levels of melatonin may contribute to migraine. As we age, our bodies produce less, so I take 5mg of melatonin two hours before bedtime. I have not experienced any side effects.

Probiotics: The gut-brain connection has become a hot topic, and it makes sense. If the gut is not happy, neither is the head. At the recommendation of a pharmacist, I take a probiotic containing 20 billion CFU (colony forming units) with breakfast. My gut works better, and this may be helping the rest of my body as my metabolism improves. The gut is called the second brain and provides direct access to the rest of our body's metabolic activities.

Hormones: I apply an estradiol patch twice weekly and swallow 100mg of progesterone each evening. Maintaining hormones at a constant level improves my sleep, eliminates hot flashes, and protects my bones. There is controversy surrounding hormone replacement, but I feel better with HRT, and I want to ward off osteoporosis. I am at risk for bone fracture because of a small frame and all-too-frequent steroid prescriptions to break up unrelenting migraine and sinus infections. Weighing one's risk factors for cancer vs. quality of life with the advice of a supportive gynecologist can help a patient make an informed decision about hormone replacement.

- Massage: I am a believer in regular massage therapy with a skilled provider. Currently I schedule a ninety-minute massage, every two weeks. DeAnne focuses on my head and neck for migraine and my lower back for pinched and complaining nerves from spinal stenosis and resulting sciatica. She works me over with her special technique she calls "bodywork," tugging on my arms and legs, "cupping" my back with small, heated bowls, digging with tools into my trigger points, massaging with heated Petoskey stones,[27] and her talented hands. I often climb gingerly onto her table pre-massage, and ninety minutes later inhabit a younger body, dancing pain-free out to my car. I wish the effects would last longer than a day or two, but everyday living seems to reknot my muscles.

Prevention is better than treatment. I exercise daily to produce a boost of natural painkiller endorphins. No side effects, and it improves my state of mind. And a positive mindset can be curative.

Sleep, lovely sleep. It is the best cure on earth if you can get it. I stay on a schedule, avoid caffeine after 3pm, no heavy meals late in the day, and utilize an unwinding ritual to put the day away. I read in bed for 30-60 minutes each night and avoid blue light from screens. An engrossing novel or work of nonfiction takes me into another world and allows me to ignore my issues. If I have a nagging thought, I write it down so I can deal with it tomorrow, rather than wrestling with it all night. Ear plugs, eye shades during full moon, and white sound from a HEPA filter block out the world for eight hours. I keep the pet out of my bed. My sixty-two-pound standard poodle sleeps in his open top crate on the floor beside me. It took two nights to get him acclimated, and he now begs for his own bed each evening. A few favored toys remain in his crate for nighttime cuddling. Three tiny Milk-bones™ signal goodnight to Vinny Van Poodle. If I cannot sleep,

I pray for others. Sometimes I consume a light snack and sip half a cup of Sleepytime or Valerian tea. A stable blood sugar wards off migraine. I meditate, though it is not so easy with ADD, and sometimes enumerate my blessings. On winter eves, I drop the thermostat to 62 degrees, don comfy sleepwear, and preheat the bed to warm my blue toes with a heating pad that runs along the foot under the bottom sheet. I usually click off this heating device before nodding off and I can sleep sockless in comfort despite Raynaud's. Cold toes will keep me awake.

An ergonomic workstation is vital for a migraineur. I have a standing desk which can be raised and lowered for comfortable typing. While standing on a rubber mat, I wear Dansko™ clogs for support, or I sit upon an Aeron® chair with a lumbar support. Moving around and out of the chair every hour is best for me and drinking water is a good reminder to take five.

Picking up a prescription at a compounding pharmacy, I speak with the pharmacist who is a fellow migraineur. Ann is approximately sixty years of age and says she has given up on prescription drugs for her migraine. She uses a TENS® unit on the nape of her neck at her first symptom, which is neck pain. She takes a cocktail of OTC remedies: caffeine, Sudafed® (pseudoephedrine HCl), naproxen, and aspirin all together. She says it works better than anything else she has tried. We all react differently to medications and since my gut can no longer tolerate nonsteroidal anti-inflammatories such as naproxen and aspirin, I will not experiment with her precise regimen. However, during my next brainstorm, I apply electrodes attached to a TENS unit to the nape of my neck after I swallow a triptan and two acetaminophen extra strength. The ensuing headache seems to be less severe than usual and of shorter duration. This neurostimulation of the occipital nerves is a distraction from pain. Some patients have gone a step further with implanted electrodes to interfere with severe pain. Less invasive is better if it works.

Ann, PharmD, says she mixes up lidocaine nasal spray for frequent migraineurs and says, "It must work. They come back for refills." I may try this next if my new script for Timolol® (beta-blocker) nasal spray does not work or gives me unpleasant side effects. I try the compounded nasal spray on a day when the first twinges of migraine occur, and I can stay at home to monitor for low blood pressure. I lay down to relax for thirty minutes after ingesting Amerge, two Tylenol extra strength tabs, and spraying the Timolol solution up both nostrils. I am cautiously optimistic as the headache recedes instead of advancing. I return to my desk, thrilled with this new-found remedy, until the hours-long roar of a neighbor's leaf blower blasts away my triumph. The brainstorm roars back, and my victory dance is premature. Peace is fragile. Since beta blockers inhibit the stimulating effect of adrenalin, they decrease electrical excitability of nerve cells. The fast-acting nasal spray is quickly absorbed and so far, is better-tolerated than an oral formulation. However, the constant drone of the neighbor's leaf blower, rattling my windows and overwhelming my sensitive neurons defeats the dose this time. I will try again. This preparation is not covered by insurance, costs about $80, and is shelf-stable for only thirty days. It is not the answer to my pain-cancelling prayers, but it is another tool.

When I was working, one of my cardiac surgeon customers, noting the frequency of my migraine headaches, suggests that I visit one of his referring cardiologists for an echocardiogram to check for a PFO. According to the American Heart Association, "a *patent foramen ovale* is a hole in the wall of tissue (septum) between the left and right upper chambers of the heart (atria). This hole is present in every human fetus to allow blood to bypass the lungs prior to birth. When a newborn enters the world and takes its first breath, the foramen ovale begins to close, and within a few months it has sealed completely in about 75% of the population. When it remains open it is called a *patent foramen ovale*, patent meaning open." This usually does not cause an issue for most patients and requires no treatment unless the patient is throwing blood clots. The procedure to close it is invasive, either by threading a patch via a catheter from the groin into the heart, or during open-heart surgery. Dr. S alerted me to the fact that whenever cardiovascular surgeons perform an open-heart procedure and discover a PFO they routinely close it. Postoperatively many patients who had previously experienced migraine report serendipitous relief after closure of PFO. Patients with aura report the best post-op relief from migraine. Since I do not experience aura with my migraine, I weigh the possible gain from the procedure versus the odds of complications from stroke, pericardial tamponade, atrial fibrillation, and death. Since I am not willing to undergo closure of PFO electively, I have not had my heart scanned for this defect.

The FDA recently approved a non-invasive vagal nerve stimulator for acute treatment of migraine. In the 1990s, while studying an implanted vagal stimulator for epilepsy seizures, researchers found that patients in the study who experienced migraine noted a reduction in the frequency of attacks. Gamma-Core®, the non-invasive device, was originally used for prevention and treatment of patients in the throes of cluster headache. Since cluster headache comprises just 1% of the headache population, researchers moved on to study the migraine population. Currently the device requires a prescription forwarded to Gamma Core. The device is leased from the manufacturer, requiring reactivation at $700 per month, while the patient attempts to receive coverage from her insurance company. There may be a month or two of "free trial" while the patient awaits approval from bean counters who decide quality of life issues such as pain management. This device is currently being studied for pregnant patients with migraine or cluster, since they should not take certain drugs. Vagal nerve stimulation quiets the brain by decreasing excitatory signals. It can affect heart rhythm and may slow heart rate. On my next neurology visit for Botox injections, I may ask my neurologist if I should consider a trial of this treatment. But since I have low blood pressure, I may not be a candidate. The device is approved for acute treatment but not for prevention since it did not meet the desired endpoint, though data trended favorably.

Cefaly, which I discuss in chapter sixteen is another nerve stimulation device approved for both prevention and treatment of acute migraine. Another approach is transcranial magnetic stimulation (TMS), which stimulates nerve cells in the brain with a magnetic field. This treatment is currently approved for migraine, chronic depression when other treatments have failed, obsessive-compulsive disorder (OCD), and to help smokers quit their habit when standard treatments are ineffective. Too bad I do not have any of these other indications since the price per symptom will go down. TMS may be an option if I get into trouble with medication over-use headache, i.e., requiring triptans and other abortive meds for three days per week or more. I have not tried TMS for my brainstorms but will watch for longer term studies.

After a recent eye exam, an optimistic optician talks me into a pair of Maui Jim rose-tinted glasses. He says they subdue his migraine. On the advice of my optometrist, I also order computer glasses, which are single vision lenses which focus on my monitor at arms-length. Craning my neck to peer up and down through progressive lenses, while searching for the sweet spot of acuity, may be contributing to migraine at my writing desk. The neck knows. It is attached to the brainstem.

Update: The rose-colored sunglasses are relaxing to wear, but on a sunny day I tried them at my desk and the monitor screen appeared black. Apparently, the lenses block out a particular blue wavelength. So, I grab a cap and pull the brim low over the computer glasses to finish my work.

chapter 21

TRIPPING ON TRIPTANS

The greater the dark, the easier to be a star.
—Jerzey Lec Stanislaw[28]

When I cannot outrun an approaching migraine, I employ artillery. My drug of choice is nearly always a triptan, unless I have used up my allotment of two-three days per week or ten doses per month, coupled with either one gram of acetaminophen and/or an antinausea drug like Compazine, and a strong cup of caffeine. One of my esteemed neurologists advises, "always take two drugs to abort migraine and take them early." If one has no underlying cardiac conditions to preclude using a vasoconstrictor, or other contraindications such as peripheral vascular disease, cerebrovascular syndromes, uncontrolled hypertension, liver disease, currently using ergot-containing medications, a few antibiotics which a pharmacist can give advice on adequate time between doses, using other 5-HT1 agonists, monoamine-oxidase-A inhibitors, or have hemiplegic or basilar migraine, triptans may abort migraine if taken early. Various triptan formulations have differing half-lives, i.e. how long a drug remains active, and routes of administration which determine time to relief. Triptans are in the class of drugs called serotonin 5-HT1 receptor agents. They inhibit excessive dilation of cerebral arteries.

Caution: I learned first-hand that triptans can cause medication overuse headache (MOH) if used too often. I spent a week as an inpatient trying to climb out of this slippery ditch. They can also trigger serotonin syndrome if co-administered with SSRIs, TCAs, and MAO inhibitors. Serotonin syndrome is a serious drug reaction that can be life threatening. A build-up of serotonin in high concentration will present with warning signals according to the Mayo Clinic of "agitation, insomnia, confusion, rapid heart rate, high blood pressure, dilated pupils, loss of muscle coordination, twitching muscles, high blood pressure, muscle rigidity, heavy sweating, diarrhea, headache, shivering, goose bumps, high fever, tremor, seizures, irregular heartbeat, unconsciousness. If you suspect you might have serotonin syndrome after starting a new drug or increasing the dose of a drug you are already using, call your health care provider right away and/or go to the emergency room. If you have severe or rapidly worsening symptoms, seek emergency treatment immediately."

Now that I have frightened you with that warning, here are some options to consider.

U.S. available triptans:

1. Almotriptan malate: Axert® 6.25mg or 12.5mg tablet; mean half-life of 3-4 hours.

2. Eletriptan hydrobromide: Relpax® 20mg or 40mg tablets, mean half-life 13 hours.

3. Frovatriptan succinate: Frova 2.5mg tablet; mean half-life of 26 hours.

4. Naratriptan: Amerge 1mg and 2.5mg tablet; half-life 6 hours.

5. Rizatriptan benzoate: Maxalt® 5mg and 10mg tablet, and Maxalt-MLT 10mg an orally disintegrating tablet; 2-3-hour half-life.

6. Sumatriptan succinate: Imitrex 25mg, 50mg, 100mg tablets; half-life of 2.5 hours, also available as Imitrex injection 4mg and 6mg pen, subcutaneous administration and Imitrex nasal spray.

7. Zolmitriptan: Zomig® 5mg tablet 3-hour half-life, and Zomig nasal spray.

If one cannot take triptans, some of the newer monoclonal antibodies may be useful as migraine abortives, in addition to use as preventatives. Gepants, such as Nurtec®, work to block CGRP, as well as Lasmiditan®, a serotonin receptor agonist; Reyvow®, brand name in a class called ditans and related to triptans, as well as anti-inflammatories: aspirin, ibuprofen, naproxen, diclofenac; ergots, such as DHE-45 and Migranal, isometheptine, and anti-emetics which may take the edge off pain in addition to treating nausea. Acetaminophen, one gram works for me at times. And I find that ice on the head, while lying in a dark room under a blanket often provides the most reliable relief. Brain freeze? I prefer homemade peach or strawberry-rhubarb gelato. If I am trying to sleep, I use a cold gel strip which adheres to the forehead and cools the skin with camphor as the active ingredient. It sometimes makes a difference at bedtime, distracting the pain signal and allowing me to nod off. Sweet dreams.

chapter 22

LOVING THE BUZZ

If this is coffee, please bring me some tea; but if this is tea, please bring me some coffee.
—Abraham Lincoln[29]

I need coffee strong enough to awaken my ancestors.
—Unknown

Life is too short to drink bad coffee.
—Susan P. Ryan

I admit that I love coffee, tea, and dark chocolate, all delivering tasty doses of the most widely consumed psychoactive substance, caffeine. Through trial and error, I find that keeping my doses on schedule is the key to safely enjoy this simple pleasure. I have reduced my habit to a maximum of three cups per day, starting with a generous scoop of freshly ground dark roast in a brown paper filter, pouring boiling water over a single dose with breakfast. I often sprinkle cinnamon onto the coffee before hot water for a boost in flavor and antioxidants, and the reported positive effect of maintaining blood sugar levels. I repeat with lunch, sometimes lunching early to get to that second cup. I believe that less caffeine may be absorbed if consumed with food. And coffee's high level of antioxidants may reduce inflammation in the body, which is a hallmark of pain. In the afternoon I sometimes brew a third cup but often enjoy tea, either hot or iced, Irish or green. I watch the clock and do my utmost to finish caffeine consumption by 3 pm to protect my sleep. Ingesting the same amount each day at the same time is vital to avoiding a caffeine withdrawal headache. Caffeine's half-life is six hours, which means that a 4 pm espresso will be reduced to half of its potency by 10 pm. A half cup of java at 10 pm as a nightcap is equivalent to a full shot at 4 pm. In ten hours, all caffeine will be cleared.

Another favorite is a steamy Americano. Though while I have enjoyed my espresso machine for many years, I read a study which shows that unfiltered coffee causes elevated LDL, low density lipoprotein levels in the blood. Since I have high cholesterol, I have switched to the pour over method with an unbleached paper or bamboo filter. My cholesterol has dropped a bit, though that may be partially due to the statin my internist insists I need. My French press is also banished to the back of the pantry since diterpenes (oils) from coffee beans are the culprit. These oils are mostly captured on coffee filters.

My Irish grandmother introduced me to the pleasure of afternoon tea. We sat in her soft upholstered chairs in a sunroom on a bluff overlooking Lake Huron, beside her stacks of books and newspapers, sipping tea from blue ceramic cups on saucers, poured from a matching teapot. There may have been biscuits, but I remember the strong black tea and how it warmed me after hours of beachcombing in the wind.

Katherine Tallmadge, MA, RD, LD, spokesperson for the American Diabetic Association says, "There doesn't seem to be a downside to tea. First tea has less caffeine. It's pretty well established that the compounds in tea, their flavonoids, are good for the heart and may reduce cancer." Green, white, and black tea are loaded with antioxidants, as well as "caffeine and theanine which affect the brain and heighten alertness."

The ADA lists benefits of tea consumption:[30]

1. Green tea's antioxidants may interfere with the growth of bladder, breast, lung, stomach, pancreatic, and colorectal cancers; prevent clogging of the arteries, burn fat, counteract oxidative stress on the brain, reduce the risk of neurological disorders like Alzheimer's and Parkinson's diseases; reduce the risk of stroke, and improve cholesterol levels.

2. Caffeine has been linked to a decreased risk for chronic illness such as cardiovascular disease, Type II diabetes, Parkinson's Disease, gallstones, and some cancers.

3. Black tea may protect lungs from damage caused by exposure to cigarette smoke. It may also reduce the risk of stroke.

4. One study showed that white tea has the most potent anticancer properties compared to more processed teas.

Herbal teas are my evening sipping choice since they contain no caffeine. There have been fewer studies on herbal teas, but the ADA lists some findings: *Chamomile may help prevent complications from diabetes, like loss of vision and nerve and kidney damage, and stunt the growth of cancer cells. Hibiscus may lower blood pressure.* Celestial Seasons Sleepytime™, Traditional Medicinals Organic Nighty Night Extra™ (valerian), peppermint, Stash Lemon-Ginger™, and Tazo Sweet Orange™ are favorites in my pantry after three pm. And a special treat is Stash Decaf Chai Spice™, with a splash of whole milk for a tasty Chai Latte.

According to the Harvard TH Chan School of Public Health, "In moderation, caffeine may be considered a healthy drink. It is a source of Vitamin B-2, magnesium, and polyphenols." Physiologically, caffeine increases levels of alertness, increases energy, ability to concentrate, and may improve athletic performance. Negative effects from too much caffeine include anxiety, increased heart rate, insomnia, and restlessness.

Dark chocolate contains caffeine and beta-phenylethylamine which are both vasoconstrictors. Though chocolate is considered a trigger for some poor migraineurs, it may also be a treatment during an acute brainstorm. A study published in *The Journal of Ethnopharmacology* in 2008: "Repression of calcitonin gene-related peptide expression in trigeminal neurons by a Theobroma cacao extract" by Marcie J. Abbey, Vinit V. Patil, Carrie V. Vause, and Paul L. Durham[31] shows in a rat-model how this extract from chocolate may block trigeminal nerve firing, a likely location for migraine initiation. This is very similar to the pharmacological action of a class of new, expensive CGRP inhibiting drugs which are improving the lives of many chronic migraine sufferers.

A simple square (or two) of dark chocolate, especially with nuts and sea salt, is oh so heavenly to savor with my afternoon coffee or tea. Some patients may crave chocolate prior to migraine and are convinced that chocolate is their trigger. But how could something so lovely be triggering? Perhaps these patients are simply chocolate deficient. I believe that dosage is the key. Just the right amount may tamp down a headache in its infancy. I am a bit of a chocolate snob ever searching for high quality chocolate. It is less expensive than most pharmaceuticals and my only caution is to avoid over-consumption, since the accompanying sugar will impact blood glucose levels, and the resultant drop after a large dose may be enough to trigger a rebound headache. Moderation in dosage is key to enjoying this treatment.

Caffeine has been implicated as causing migraine due to its vasoconstrictive and diuretic properties. It has also been used in many headache medications for these very effects. Many headache drugs are vasoconstrictors with diuretic properties, but none of them have the flavor and pleasant attributes of coffee enjoyed with a friend or a good book. When I feel a headache coming on, I usually grab my coffee cup and a square of dark chocolate along with two Tylenol Extra Strength tabs. If I lie down with ice on my head immediately afterwards, I sometimes find that my headache has drifted off and I may enjoy thirty minutes of rest. The trick is in the timing. I must ingest caffeine at the first hint of migraine and lay down before caffeine's energizing effects kick in. If I fall asleep for thirty minutes, I may wake up feeling refreshed and pain-free. It is worth a try if I am at home. And it is a tasty treatment.

A February 19, 2024 article in Medscape Medical News states: "Habitual consumption of caffeine is not associated with frequency, duration, or intensity of episodic migraines, a new study showed. Investigators said the findings suggest caffeine restrictions in migraineurs may not be necessary."[32] **Caveat: Avoid caffeine powders.** According to the FDA, a teaspoonful of pure caffeine or highly concentrated caffeine is equivalent to about **twenty-eight cups of coffee.** That dose will be a most unpleasant and hazardous way to get in touch with one's nocturnal side.

chapter 23

BALANCE YOUR 'LYTES AND DIM THE LIGHTS

The cure for anything is salt water: sweat, tears, or the sea.
—Karen Blixen[33]

Fed up with pharmaceutical side effects which are as life-interrupting as migraine, I decide to retry a strategy that biologically and chemically makes sense. The Academy of Nutrition and Dietetics estimates that "about 75% of Americans are in a state of chronic dehydration... even a subtle dehydration of 2% can trigger fatigue, headaches, difficulty concentrating, lightheadedness, and more." So, if this paucity of hydration is the number one cause of migraine, how can one rehydrate neurons (brain cells) effectively? Plain water seems to run through me like an open faucet during a migraine episode. I find myself racing to the loo on the hour.

During these sieges I add an envelope of powdered electrolytes to my water bottle to stem the tide, but after I re-read "Fighting the Migraine Epidemic: How to Treat and Prevent Migraine Without Medicines, An Insider's View" by Angela A. Stanton, Ph.D., I decide to test her system on a more rigorous basis. Dr. Stanton's field of expertise is neuroscience and decision-making. She is a long-term migraineur who claims significant relief by keeping her brain adequately hydrated.

When we are dehydrated, there is an electrolyte imbalance, which does not allow our brain cells to retain enough water for healthy functioning. Our neurons are thirsting for a solution of potassium and sodium in a ratio of 2:1. This can be accomplished by assaying one's food and maintaining this equilibrium. Websites and/or dietitians can help you analyze your diet for these vital salts. Once you understand which foods are high in sodium and potassium, you can begin to balance your intake and placate your neurons. For instance, if I eat a green salad, which is high in potassium, I make sure to sprinkle a dose of sea salt (sodium chloride) on it. As we age, we are cautioned to watch our salt intake to keep blood pressure under control. But high blood pressure is not universal. Dr. Stanton avers that most migraineurs have low blood pressure though I have not seen a scientific breakdown on this. Since my blood pressure is quite low, I find that adding a bit of sodium to my food usually perks me up as it balances my diet of daily leafy green potassium-rich foods. However, if you are a migraineur with hypertension or kidney disease, please consult with your physician or a nutritionist before embarking on this electrolyte balancing journey.

My on-call powder packets contain a higher quantity of

potassium relative to sodium. The ratio is not exactly 2:1, but it is in the ballpark, and this hydration seems to help me. On days when I may be vulnerable to brainstorm, I dissolve an electrolyte packet into sixteen ounces of water once, twice, or three times during the day. So far, only one migraine during three weeks of paying closer attention to this balance, despite see-sawing barometric pressures with thunderstorms rolling in from Lake Michigan and assaulting my brain and sinuses. Since hot weather is another migraine trigger for me, I was thrilled to spend a recent afternoon kayaking with temperatures in the mid 80s and my brain uncomplaining. It is early in this experiment, and with loads of overly sensitive neurons to keep hydrated and perhaps retrained, the jury is still out. Without any perceptible side-effects for me at this point, I am optimistic that I may have found a worthwhile and easy treatment.

Useful for me: Dr. Price's Electrolyte Mix™ contains 330mg potassium/200mg sodium. Since potassium is not a pleasant flavor, Lemon-Lime and Raspberry are both decent masking additions with stevia leaf as sweetener at 5 calories per serving. I recently ordered Electrolyte Recovery Plus Lemonade Replenishment™. This potion has zero calories, many vitamins, and 250mg potassium/110mg sodium. This flavor comes in third for me, but it is wonderful to have three choices.

I downed gallons of Gatorade™ while I was cycling in Louisville summers, but no longer, since it is loaded with sugar which unbalances me. The company's website offers a range of electrolytes: potassium:78-195mg/L and sodium and 460-690mg/L, not ideal for my sensitive brain. Pedialyte™ contains no sugar but the inverse of a best ratio with 130mg potassium/240mg sodium.

Pedialyte Electrolyte Water Zero Sugar™ contains artificial sweeteners which may startle the fragile neurons of a migraineur's brain. It is important to read labels to learn what may be helpful or possibly triggering for your own brain.

During a recent visit with a neurologist and fellow migraineur, I shared my new-found electrolyte wisdom. Doc said, "This makes sense. When I was in medical school, I found myself craving salty corn chips just before a headache erupted." If you pay attention to your body, you may discover what it needs.

My sensitive eyes may require sunglasses on cloudy days, and sometimes indoors if overhead lights are flickering, are the wrong color temperature, or otherwise irritating. When I moved into my newest home, I changed out every single light fixture, achieving a more soothing glow, with LED lights replacing incandescent bulbs in lamps and overhead can lights. This creates a calmer atmosphere for my brain than the original stark lighting. Incremental and non-invasive steps add up to a more soothing environment for a sensitive migraine brain.

chapter 24

Pain Is Solitary

As sickness is the greatest misery, so the greatest misery of sickness is solitude.
—John Donne[34]

Five years ago, I moved forty-five miles north to a new home perched on a sandy dune, where the breeze from Lake Michigan shakes acorns from oaks and hammers my roof. Reverberating like a hailstorm though the sun is shining, this manna from heaven creates a squirrel and chipmunk haven. Hummingbirds and Monarch Butterflies flit around this idyll during warm months, and the number of deer per square mile may be greater than humans. A standard poodle puppy is my new shadow, but I have no one to cook for, few visitors, and less opportunities to get out and socialize. Moving from a small town to a more rural area just before the pandemic has isolated me more than I anticipated. While all-too-frequent migraine keeps me close to home, I feel blessed in my comfortable retreat. When my companion, Vinny Van Poodle, finally achieves gentleman manners, life may be nearly perfect except for pain and occasional loneliness. As an extrovert, I am surprised to find myself in this situation. Change happens in increments, but the realization does not always keep up, and this new life phase feels odd, unexpected. I plod along, counting good days on fingers and painful days on fingers and toes. What was once a singular chronic condition, becomes complicated by a secondary one, degenerative spine. That is a hell of a diagnosis for someone who thinks she is still young and able to do everything herself.

After dinner I walk with Vinny Van to the lake for a game of Frisbee™ at the shoreline. The beach stairs seem steeper and longer each time. We play until the poodle has slurped up his fill of sand and water and the sun creeps toward Milwaukee, melting into Big Blue. Back home, I try to hold onto a riled-up fifty-seven-pound puppy in the dark while wrangling a hose to rinse his feet and undercarriage. It is not working for either of us. I open the garage door and try to coax the agile pup to leap into the utility tub, using his sandy Frisbee and tennis balls as bait. "Not tonight," he demurs. Tony, the K-9 trainer, says: "Vinny will gain confidence for this task as he matures." Meanwhile I grab his writhing, furry body and hoist him into the tub and wonder why I did not choose a smaller companion. My last poodle was a retirement gift from my sister Mendy, and I was fifteen years younger at the time. Oh well, if this one is adequately trained, he will (maybe next year) leap into the tub, flip on the faucet, and shampoo his own curly locks.

I cancel a tee time for tomorrow. I have not played golf since I moved, and I have been looking forward to finding a new group of golf pals. But my aging back, burdened by canine dead lifts, household maintenance, yardwork, and gravity has impaired my former flexibility. I am now hesitant to swing a club and feel forced to listen to my body since it is complaining most of the time. Maybe I will become accustomed to the noise and work through back pain as I learned to work through migraine. Popping acetaminophen for the aches has provided some relief though I am no longer able to take aspirin, naproxen, ibuprofen, or prescription NSAIDs due to stomach erosion caused by frequent use for headache. But now, daily use of acetaminophen has raised a new wrinkle for me. After a month of unabated migraine, I realize that my nightly use of acetaminophen for sciatica is causing rebound headaches. As soon as each dose wears off, a headache blooms. My brain has become habituated to this regular dose and cries "more." I consume another round of steroids to break up the headache, but before I finish a methylprednisolone taper, the headache returns. Ding, ding, ding. I am still taking the damn acetominophen at bedtime for my back, which whines and wakes me up whenever I roll over in bed. What fresh hell is this?

My friend Rose is often inhabited by pain from rheumatoid arthritis. "She's back," says Rose as she names her pain. "The bitch is back, and she moves from hands to feet, to back, to knees." The unwelcome guest does not sign Rose's lodger ledger and comes and goes as she pleases. What shall I name my pain in the brain?

Storm. Susan's Storm. We coexist, though not willingly on my part. I pray for relief and search for banishment of my storm.

I make an appointment with a neurologist who prescribes a lidocaine patch which I apply to the L-4—S-1 inflamed area at bedtime. It has been four weeks, and I am sleeping slightly better with this new palliative. When my hips feel tight and achy from this spinal issue, despite stretching, I apply cannabis cream or roll on Penetrex®, a homeopathic balm, and occasionally I apply Voltaren® (diclofenac sodium), a topical NSAID gel and gain another few degrees of relief.

So now that I have the diagnosis of the number one cause of disability, chronic lower back pain, along with the number two cause of disability, chronic migraine, I trudge on, trying to manage immediate pain without causing the submerged pain to flare up. Physical therapy stretches each morning calm the back beast but are not curative. Poodle hikes are distracting and get me outside. Although my podiatrist warns that my five-seven miles of hiking each day are causing a recurrence of plantar fasciitis as he jabs three cortisone injections into my right heel and tapes the foot for support. My canine companion provides structure, a bit of comfort, and a lightness in my life. There is unpredictability while living with pain and I find relief in novel ways. On the days that I am on the sofa, with ice on my head, I toss the ball to the pooch again and again and again. He gives me a reason to weather the storm.

chapter 25

NOT YOUR MOTHER'S HEAVY METAL

I was looking for something a lot heavier, yet melodic at the same time. Something different from heavy metal, a different attitude.
—Kurt Cobain[35]

A very light metal, less dense than aluminum, magnesium is the fourth most abundant mineral in the human body and migraineurs should be interested in the basic chemistry of this vital nutrient. To be absorbed from the gastrointestinal tract, it must be attached to another molecule, hence the many forms of magnesium available on the shelf of your local vitamin emporium. Since this nutrient is excreted via the kidneys, and through sweat, I have become proactive in replenishing magnesium that is flushed out during migraine with those oh-so-frequent bathroom breaks or during a sweaty activity. Alcohol, hypertension, diabetes, loop diuretics, proton-pump inhibitors, and antacids also hasten the excretion of magnesium.

Many physicians recommend magnesium oxide supplementation for migraine prophylaxis. This is not an especially well-absorbed form, but it may work for some. Other forms with better absorption are magnesium malate, -glycinate, -taurate, -lactate, -citrate, -chloride, -aspartate, and -threonate. There are fewer side effects with magnesium than most potions prescribed for migraine, but certain individuals should use caution, such as those with impaired kidney function. A physician or pharmacist can provide individual dosage recommendations and monitor possible interactions with other meds such as antibiotics, diuretics, muscle relaxers, and cardiac drugs. Dietary intake of magnesium is the best way to supplement. Look for fresh foods that provide high levels of magnesium such as almonds, avocado, bananas, black beans, dairy, dark chocolate (yes!), lentils, oily fish such as tuna and mackerel, peanuts, seeds, spinach, whole wheat, and more. If you ingest too much magnesium, diarrhea will be your clue. I have experimented with different formulas of magnesium with varying results. Living with IBS, my gut is super sensitive and does not always tolerate oral magnesium. But when my gut is quiet, I sneak in this supplement once, twice, or three times per day and I feel that it tempers the migraine monster. Even when serum magnesium levels are within normal range, nerve cells may not contain sufficient magnesium. I am currently taking 200mg of Magnesium Glycinate three times each day. I have used other forms of magnesium and switch around according to my current tolerance. Each migraineur can experiment to find her own best tolerated and effective formulation, which is one that your body will absorb.

Why bother? Because nerve function is dependent on magnesium and nerves are truly the root of pain. I once showed up without an appointment at 5 pm on a Friday in my doctor's office. I was in the throes of a killer migraine after an unsuccessful visit to a chiropractor. This kind complementary medicine physician offered me two choices: two+ hours in a hyperbaric chamber (HBOT, hyperbaric oxygen treatment) or IV magnesium. I regret now that I did not try option A (for its novelty), which is used for treating decompression sickness in scuba divers.

It was rumored that the late Michael Jackson slept regularly in a hyperbaric chamber, but it apparently did not enhance his lifespan. According to the Mayo Clinic, "Hyperbaric oxygen therapy involves breathing pure oxygen in a pressurized environment. In a hyperbaric oxygen chamber, the pressure is increased two to three times higher than normal pressure." The theory is that your lungs will suck up more oxygen than at atmospheric pressure, and your blood ferrying the extra O2 throughout the body may "stimulate the release of growth factors and stem cells." It is plausible to test this exotic remedy, but since it was so late in the day, I opted for the rapid treatment. I did not want to detain the doctor and his staff for an extra two hours. I also wanted immediate relief.

A nurse ran a small bag of intravenous magnesium sulfate over a few minutes into my depleted body. During the infusion I felt flushed, hot, and dizzy, while fading from consciousness. I lowered my head between my knees to increase blood pressure. While I recovered from this vasovagal episode, my migraine evaporated. Poof! The blissful respite lasted for about forty-five minutes, and the headache roared back while I prepared dinner at home. I was clearly disappointed but realized that such a pronounced reaction was worth further investigation. It was evident that the bolus of magnesium was sufficient to abort a vicious brain attack, but my magnesium blood level dropped quickly since my body was using up and/or excreting magnesium rapidly. A more sustained level of magnesium is required to deter migraine. So, eat your spinach and consider an oral magnesium supplement if you have no contraindications.

A warm bath loaded with Epsom salts is a soothing way to take in magnesium. I toss in a few handfuls, as much as the volume of water will dissolve. Magnesium sulfate is absorbed through the skin and aids in relaxation of muscles. It is a perfect treat before bedtime to enhance sleep and it may ward off a headache. If fighting a current migraine, I go full Monty: an Epsom salts soak while icing my cranium. My theory is that the ice will constrict blood vessels in the head, and blood will be drawn away from the painful cranium toward the lower body. I take extra care exiting the tub after this warm glow treatment since my blood pressure may be lowered. If feeling dizzy, I drain the tub before I stand up so that I may cool off gradually as I regain a bit of blood pressure.

I am thrilled to find that topical magnesium chloride salt spray instantly relieves muscle cramps, and I share this potion with friends who have also experienced quick relief. At my suggestion, three friends applied magnesium cream before bedtime to their lower limbs and they all said this made a difference in their Restless Legs Syndrome. I keep a bottle at bedside for middle of the night charley horses following over-exertion or after wearing new shoes. A slight change of arch is enough to throw sensitive me into nocturnal leg cramps. Sometimes I apply magnesium to my temples and neck during a migraine and fall asleep more easily. I recently began to apply magnesium cream to the soles of my feet at bedtime and find that I sleep more soundly and recall vivid dreams. I will continue to experiment with topical magnesium for acute pain and sleep enhancement in addition to daily oral magnesium supplements for migraine prophylaxis. I have experienced no side effects from topical magnesium.

chapter 26

FOREST BATHING

And into the forest I go—to lose my mind and
find my soul.
—John Muir[36]

And I may lose my headache while I amble outside and
hug a tree.
—Susan P. Ryan

Wearing sunglasses and a hat on bright days and dressed for the weather, I inhale my free dose of fresh air. When I feel a migraine sneaking up on me, it often recedes when I step through the doorway and head to the park. Immersion in the natural environment is without side effects and may be just what I need. On migraine days, my walks are shorter than the grand hikes my standard poodle prefers, but they are beneficial. From behind dark glasses I notice blades of grass, waving branches, flittering leaves, delicate wildflowers, buzzy insects, and chattering birds while I ramble. It is not hyperbaric oxygen, but my body feels enlivened by fresh air especially on cooler days.

"In 1990 the Japanese Ministry of Agriculture, Forestry, and Fisheries coined the term Shinrin-yoku which translates roughly as forest bathing." ~Allison Aubrey, NPR 7/17/14, Morning Edition report "Forest Bathing: A Retreat to Nature Can Boost Immunity and Mood."[37]

A day stuck inside with migraine is stifling, while an hour breathing fresh air eases whatever ails me, except hay fever. It inspires new ways of dealing with chronic pain. A decent distraction is the best method I have found to ignore pain and being outdoors is my favorite remedy. If I am feeling particularly lousy, I simply sit on the patio wearing a hat and sunglasses, sipping water. My slower pace directs a sharper focus on the natural world. And while I am oh-so-still, a green and ruby hummingbird sits on my arm for a brief visit. Sometimes after I pick up a rake, a hose, or the dog's leash, the migraine tiptoes off stage.

Sunny Fitzgerald writes in *National Geographic*, October 18, 2019: "The Secret to Mindful Travel: "A Walk in the Woods." She offers curated forest bathing locales: Adirondack Mountains of New York, Costa Rica, New Zealand, Kenya, and Hawai`i.[38]

I can vouch for the exquisite forest bathing in Costa Rica's rainforests, floating on New Zealand's Milford Sound, and cycling around Hawai`i's Big Island, but for now, I find equal inspiration closer to home. A quiet green space is a sensory indulgence. I lean against a tree for strength. Trickling water is delicious to my ears and the roar of Lake Michigan soothes my body and soul with a rush of negative ions. Closing my eyes and breathing deeply, I relax in nature's healing embrace.

Biophilia, according to Merriam-Webster©, is *the human tendency to interact or be closely associated with other forms of life in nature. Filia is from the Greek, meaning friendship, a love for, tendency toward, or excessive appetite or craving for.* My personal filia: surrounded by blue spruce in the snow and floating on or hiking beside moving water in any season. Sneaking up on blue herons and snapping turtles is a spring, summer, and fall diversion from pain while paddling my kayak. Being outdoors contributes to feelings of well-being, by lowering stress and anxiety. Swimming or walking at an easy pace quiets my over-active brain. Lingering outdoors is a simple, non-invasive treatment, without side effects, and it lightens my load.

chapter 27

MOVE YOUR BODY, EASE YOUR MIND

The chief function of the body is to carry the brain around.
—Thomas Edison[39]

When I belonged to the Louisville Bicycle Club and spent hours each week pumping up and gliding down verdant hills in Kentucky, the chunky monkey neurologist, who was treating me for migraine, suggested that I "go outside and get some exercise." Huh? A few times each week I joined group rides of fifteen to one hundred miles and was in the best physical condition of my adult life. But heat and humidity triggered migraine. This so-called headache expert prescribed a few drugs off-label for migraine prevention which precipitated my heat intolerance and increased my summer headache frequency. When I retired and moved to

Michigan, the psychologist on staff at a headache institute told me to back off on intense exercise and steered me to yoga and walking, with breathing exercises designed to slow me down. Since I was newly retired from a high energy job of selling heart valves in four states, my lifestyle change was like driving at the speed of the pace car at the Indy 500 and trying to merge into a 15-mph school zone. Always active, I find it difficult to sit still even during brainstorm. I power through it, rarely taking time off to recover and renew. This may be why the monthly episodic brainstorms eventually transformed to chronic migraine.

With early retirement at fifty-five, I have enjoyed the past fifteen years without the demands of a real job, though I still pushed myself the first several years by attending graduate school and completing a Master of Fine Arts in writing program. Compared to my undergraduate science courses in pharmacy school and my stressful job as a heart valve specialist for Medtronic, graduate school was a walk in the woods. And writing is a tonic for me since writing and walking are interconnected. I need to walk each day to sort my thoughts before writing. On hot days I head out early. In winter, I bundle up and hike after lunch. Tiptoe, if necessary, between raindrops, but I am outside to offer my brain fresh air and inspiration. Regular exercise can be a preventative measure for migraineurs. After exercise, plasma levels of beta-endorphin, endocannabinoid, and neurotrophic factors increase, all natural antidepressants without the side effects of pharmaceuticals. An individual's migraine-triggering threshold may be reset by regular exercise, resulting in a lower frequency of attacks, though running a marathon after months of pain-provoked sofa-surfing is not advised. Intense exercise without proper conditioning will trigger my brainstorm.

My sister Mary Ellen gave me the perfect retirement gift: a standard poodle puppy. Ella Fitz Poodle nagged me to walk every day regardless of the weather or what may be on my schedule. I became a hiker, and my bicycle tires flattened from lack of use. I began to see the world at a slower pace, on poodle time, every day without fail. Walking each day is vital for my health. Being outdoors tunes me into nature and I have met loads of people on my walkabouts that I would not have met otherwise. Walking with a sturdy canine companion is a preferred treatment for whatever ails me.

My newest pup, Vinny Van Poodle is a gentleman-in-training and is not yet up to Ella's best-dog-ever gold standard, but he gets me outside each day. He is my hiking buddy, and he is learning to deal with my brainstorm. Some days he is a gem, and other days he wears an E-collar which reminds him with a gentle buzz to use his inside voice. It is soothing to have a furry companion during pain, and I will be grateful when Vinny assumes his role as migraine therapy dog.

chapter 28

NOT SO TRIGGER-HAPPY

A gem cannot be polished without friction, nor a man perfected without trials.
—Lucius Annaeus Seneca[40]

Oh, to be a diamond in the rough, to avoid battering brainstorms.
—Susan P. Ryan

Living beside Lake Michigan, with weather fronts rolling in upon white caps, I sometimes wonder why I decided to retire here. It is lovely until the barometric pressure roller coasters and sets my head off on a multi-day migraine odyssey. For these trips, I keep ice packs on call in the freezer to numb my sensitive skull along with chilled ear plugs, in an attempt to chill as close to the brain as possible. Living in the fruit-belt near Lake Michigan, I have found tasty treatments while inspecting the glorious bounty of the Holland farmers' market. The mountains of fragrant, fresh fruit make my mouth water, and I decide to create a diversion for my pain. Homemade strawberry-rhubarb gelato is my favorite placebo, with Red Haven Peach gelato a close second. Third, is coffee gelato with dark chocolate shavings. Returning from a semester residency of writing in Italy, I bought a gelato-maker and often churn out small batches when local fruits are at their peak. In a pinch I toss frozen peaches and blueberries into a blender with Greek yogurt, a splash of tart cherry juice, and a dash of Saigon cinnamon for a soothing smoothie. This frozen margarita substitute quells my queasy stomach, and the chill numbs my palate and possibly the trigeminal nerve (which innervates the face, mouth, and TMJ), which is said to ignite during migraine. And a dose of protein from the dairy perks me up.

On the golf course during hot weather, I keep a wet microfiber cloth in a cooler, draping it over my neck as the temperature rises, while chugging icy electrolytes. Finding a way to navigate through pain is preferrable to missing out on everything. Be the boss. Since sciatica has crept into my sacroiliac-L5 joint, I have switched from twice-weekly rounds of golf to kayaking while I can still climb in and out of my small craft. With an adjustable seat back and moveable foot pegs, I paddle comfortably for hours, meeting mergansers and leaping bass while drifting through a watery dreamscape. Wearing a wide-brimmed hat to protect my sensitive head and prescription sunglasses, I schedule my outings for morning or early evening to avoid the hottest hours. During the pandemic, I installed a rowing machine in my library. It is useful on rainy days, during winter, and as a blood-pumping intermezzo during desk days. My road bike is set up on a trainer beside a sliding glass door so I can cycle within view of evergreens without getting too hot, too cold, or too wet. With a book rack attached to the handlebars, I read for an hour, check emails, return phone calls, or get pumped by watching a video of *le Tour de France*. One must always dream and do something aerobic each day. I try not to go overboard on my non-migraine days, but it is hard after missing out on so many days of play.

Since sinus pain is akin to migraine, I manage my year-round allergies with daily allergy drops, a nightly antihistamine, a monthly grooming appointment for my non-shedding pet, nasal irrigation as needed, and avoidance of smoke and air pollution. Strong perfumes, the laundry aisle of the grocery store, and air fresheners are not my friends. Scented and even paraffin non-scented candles are unwelcome, since they spew out petrochemicals as they combust. I have a HEPA filter running continuously in my bedroom for improved air quality and I change the furnace filter regularly while maintaining the humidity in the house at a comfortable level year-round. I adjust my space and life for a more peaceful brain.

At the suggestion of my allergist, I raise the head of my bed by six inches, hiring a couple of strong men to lift and position the king-sized sleigh bed onto two blocks. The first few nights are challenging as I awake often to find myself sliding off my pillow and toward the end of the bed. And the height of the bed is a bit daunting in the middle of the night as I try to vault into it after a trip to the loo in the dark. One December night I find myself barreling down the luge run in nearby Muskegon, bouncing against the walls of the course as my sled hits sixty miles per hour. Powered by an adrenalin surge, I awake to a blast of Michigan winter ruffling my nightie and frosting my nose. Heading to the kitchen for a glass of water, I find the patio door blown open by a gale off Lake Michigan, with sleet slanting onto the slate floor. My dreams are often vivid imitations of life.

The radically inclined bed seems to help my breathing and lessens overnight drainage which Dr. Reddy attributes to chronic sinusitis and silent GERD. He tells me that the valve between the stomach and esophagus does not close completely as we age, with stomach acid entering the esophagus, which is not lined with an acid-tolerating surface like that of the stomach. This esophageal irritation can incite the sinuses to secrete mucus to protectively coat the esophagus. Ding. It makes sense that I have been choking on drainage for several months, interfering with my sleep, a contributing trigger for increased migraine. I agree to reduce my intake of acidic and spicy foods, limit my intake of caffeine, and consume smaller meals, with an earlier dinner time. Doc tells me to wear loose-fitting clothes to prevent squeezing the stomach. No more Spanx® and sleek outfits. Age has its disappointments and privileges.

My next stop is an otolaryngologist who is pleased to hear about my radical bed head raising, frequent neti pot usage, and other measures I use to tamp down allergies. He adds a new expensive, non-formulary nasal spray, Ipratropium Bromide®, along with a more powerful flushing system for my head: NeilMed Sinus Rinse®, which feels like a firehouse compared to the gentle rinsing of the neti pot. Fingers crossed as I work with this new regimen, careful not to use it late in the day or I experience residual saline drainage whenever I roll over in bed. Clearer sinuses should be helpful in reducing frequency of migraine.

I recently purchased a UV light which I position on my nightstand when I strip the bed each week for cleaning. Using a remote control, I turn on this light for sixty minutes after removing houseplants and pet. I close the door and allow the sterilizing light to kill dust mites, a top allergen. A bit of ozone lingers after the timer stops and I air out the room. Since implementing this latest tweak, I am breathing a bit easier and sleeping more soundly. Incremental steps add up and promote healing.

chapter 29

Eat Right for **Your** Brain

One cannot think well, love well, sleep well if one has not dined well.
—Virginia Woolf[41]

A health care provider suggests that I read the book *Eat Right for Your Type* by Peter J. Adamo, N.D. with Catherine Whitney. The authors propose that each of four blood types should follow a particular diet and lifestyle for optimal health. Science involves proving or disproving theories, and this seems like a reasonable supposition to challenge. My physician is all about testing this hypothesis with his tough to treat patients, and since I am without a better option, I board this plane.

Adamo looks at the evolutionary profile of blood and tells us that Type O is the original, oldest type. He posits: "Type A evolved with agrarian society; Type B emerged as humans migrated north into colder, harsher territories; and Type AB is a thoroughly modern adaptation, a result of intermingling of disparate groups. This evolutionary story relates directly to the dietary needs of each blood type today."[42]

After several weeks on this diet—I am Type A and prefer a Mediterranean diet—I do not find any difference in my health, including headache frequency and intensity. And since the 1996 publication, there have been no peer-reviewed studies published on this diet based on blood type. Probably not worth any more consideration.

Another caring physician runs me through an elimination diet. I am gluten-free, dairy-free, and lactose-free for three months and I am so hungry. During this experiment, I join a group of outdoor enthusiasts for a week-long cross country ski trip in the Cascade Mountains of eastern Washington. While fellow skiers consume my portion of the disallowed breadbasket, I ski twelve to twenty-five miles each day, powered by lettuce wraps. Since my metabolism is amped, I struggle to extract enough fuel from fruits, veggies, and nuts with an occasional bit of fish or meat. A piece of cheese or a lovely hunk of sour dough bread is what my body craves. My gut complains after I consume too many "protein bars" which are mostly concentrated fruit. These sugar bombs are tasty but ephemeral in nutritive benefit. I drop about twelve pounds, and my friends ask if I am embarking on a new career in modeling or am I under the care of an oncologist. I undergo a colon biopsy, and it is determined that I am not gluten-intolerant: no celiac disease. I abandon this experiment.

A renowned Chicago headache clinic prescribes a "low tyramine" diet at my first visit. Lots of forbidden foods including aged cheeses, processed cured meats, pickled & fermented foods, condiments, beer, red wine, liqueurs, beans, raw onions, chocolate, MSG, breads except sourdough, nuts, chicken liver, snow peas, ripe bananas, avocados, yogurt, and foods leftover for more than two days. Watch out for nitrites, nitrates, especially in deli meats, and sausages. No artificial sweeteners. Limit tofu and tempeh, soy products like miso, soy sauce, teriyaki sauce. Citrus limited to ½ cup per day. No more than two servings of caffeine per day. ZZZZZ

The National Headache Foundation (headaches.org) suggests a *Low-Tyramine Diet for Individuals with Headache or Migraine.*[43]

1. Eat three meals each day with a snack at night or six smaller meals throughout the day.

Avoid eating high sugar foods on an empty stomach, when excessively hungry, or in place of a meal. (This makes sense since a drop in blood sugar following the sugar spike may trigger migraine.)

All foods, especially high protein foods should be prepared and eaten fresh. Be cautious of leftovers held more than one or two days in the fridge. Freeze leftovers for longer use.

Cigarette and cigar smoke contain a multitude of chemicals that will trigger or aggravate headache. AMEN.

What is tyramine and why should migraineurs avoid it? It is a 'trace amine,' derived from the amino acid tyrosine, naturally occurring in certain foods. It may trigger migraine in sensitive individuals by causing vasoconstriction and rebound dilation of cranial vessels. Tyramine is thought to direct the adrenals (the glands atop the kidneys) to secrete the neurotransmitter norepinephrine which is a powerful vasoconstrictor. This sounds like something to avoid. I tried this diet half-heartedly in the past and have decided to revisit. Armed with *The Dizzy Cook* by Alicia Wolf, I am studying her recipes, shopping for fresh foods, while missing some of my favorite foods in exchange for more headache-free days. Ms. Wolf has been plagued with Vestibular Migraine and has shared her research in this cookbook and guide, published in 2020. Her recipes look inviting, and I will pursue this as my next cure. Fresh and healthy is always a good thing.

To counter my genetic gift of high cholesterol, I have been following a Mediterranean Diet, along with a low FODMAP diet for IBS. So, I will be skipping the Dizzy Cook's red meat dishes, as well as many of the bean-centric recipes. I also hesitate to use shallots and green onions since raw onions often provoke a monster migraine. I can live without processed and cured meats, MSG, and old food, but my life requires flavors and variety, and two or three caffeine servings each day at the same times. We are all different in our tolerances and proclivities, but this book looks like a healthy guide. It may be a great idea to look up high tyramine containing foods before the next grocery visit. Fresh is best and not missing meals is vital. If we climb out of our food ruts and eat a bit differently, we may improve our quality of life.

According to an abstract, "The metabolic face of migraine:

from pathophysiology to treatment," published in *Nature Reviews Neurology*, 2019,[44] "Glucose tolerance is impaired during migraine. Patients are vulnerable to an energy crisis because neuronal activation likely increases demand during migraine and sensory processing is abnormal during migraine." I try to avoid high sugar foods since my body is working harder during brainstorms and needs a higher-octane and longer-lasting fuel than simple-sugar. I have even cut down on my once daily dark chocolate nibble and notice an improvement in decreased migraine frequency. I now consider sugar as a special occasion treat such as birthday cake, sampling a slice of seasonal fruit pie, and a bowl of homemade peach gelato on a summer day. Cookies no longer accompany my afternoon tea, and I feel better. I enjoy nuts, navel oranges, blueberries on my breakfast oatmeal, and local fresh fruits, either in season or from my freezer. I do not feel deprived since I am experiencing less brainstorms. This worthwhile dietary change keeps my blood sugar and my brain in better balance.

MIND BRAKES

Thunder quakes.
  A gale blows and cracks trees.
    Rain torrents, floods, and overflows banks.
      Memory fails.
        Crashing waves erase words.
          Joy recedes to darkest corner.
            And I surrender to Morpheus
           to dream myself back
         to health and good cheer.
      From unconscious
    to subconscious
        I
      Float
       .
        .
       .
      .
    Trying to d-i-s-s-o-l-v-e **pain**.
   I crave refreshment to create myself anew.
  Reborn at dawn in a white gown,
 Head cradled in clouds,
Mind o-p-e-n-s to a fresh start.

            —Susan P. Ryan

chapter 30

Why Does Migraine Thrive?

The world breaks everyone, and afterward, some are stronger at the broken places.[45]
—Ernest Hemingway

Pain is a survival mechanism which activates in an unsuitable environment. Migraine may have developed from oversensitization of an early warning system. We migraineurs may be advanced on the evolutionary ladder since we are more attuned to deleterious environmental substances: the first to smell a natural gas leak, smoke, spoiled food, a predator's musk. Migraine can be protective, helping us to avoid toxins and an early demise. This allows us to reproduce, passing on our genetic proclivity, ensuring survival of the fittest, and the migraine gene. Ahem. What seems like a weakness may in fact be an advantageous trait. Since it is difficult for a migraineur to imbibe without certain pain, we may be protected from alcoholism by avoidance of this toxin.

Migraine is a disorder of sensory processing. The migraine brain has superpowers; it is super-sensitive; it over-reacts to stimuli such as light, sound, and odor in comparison with a non-migraine brain. There are ways to reduce one's heightened response to pain stimuli: SLEEP! Quality sleep is vital, since poor sleep lowers the pain threshold. In my introduction, I mention Matthew Walker's book *Why We Sleep*. Read it and sleep. It is a lullaby; a bedtime story that should be read until one learns how to sleep as the body requires. Fatigue is a marker of chronic pain and loss of sleep causes inflammation, depression, and anxiety. Pain medications and alcohol interfere with natural, healthy sleep cycles. Better sleep=fewer brainstorms. Engaging daily in gentle exercise increases muscle strength and reduces inflammation. Before embarking on a new pharmaceutical "cure," I weigh possible benefits vs. side effects.

Despite chronic migraine, I work on developing and nurturing a social network. I make plans to attend concerts, plays, and participate in courses on a nearby college campus. Volunteer in the community. Share one's talents. Staying in touch with others improves brain health. It may ward off brain shrinkage.

We enhance the health of our neurons by what we eat and drink. Nutritionally deficient food is detrimental to neurons. A nourishing diet decreases inflammation, another cause of pain. Adequate hydration allows neurons to create the required voltage necessary to push neurotransmitters along to other neurons. When neurons are stressed, due to lack of proper hydration, they will signal pain, MIGRAINE in susceptible individuals.

High levels of cortisol, the stress hormone, can cause epigenetic changes, permanently altering neurotransmitter switches. Sustained high levels of stress may be a reason why acute migraine becomes transformed to chronic migraine. If we dump stress, we will endure less head pain.

In a 2023 book, *The Microstress Effect*, by Rob Cross and Karen Dillon,[46] the authors state that "microstress is hard to spot because it is hard baked into our daily lives. And often it arrives through the people closest to us, making it more difficult to either admit or avoid." And since "our brains are wired to respond to conventional forms of stress, they can identify the threat and use the extra oomph of our fight-or-flight mechanisms to deal with the impact. But microstresses are too fleeting to register, especially for successful people who have learned to routinely overcome obstacles." This resonates with me. I thrived on stress during my career. Life or death was possible every day during cardiac surgery. "Like most familiar forms of stress, microstressors can increase our blood pressure and heart rate, or trigger hormonal or metabolic changes." Being more subtle, sneaky microstressors are harder to detect, but they are certainly migraine triggers. The authors recommend "actively removing even a few negative interactions ... to improve our overall well-being." The prescription of the book is "to tame microstress by nurturing connections with a variety of social groups. These contacts can be centered around athletic pursuits, volunteer work, civic or religious communities, book or dinner clubs, and so on—as opposed to close friends and family who are more likely to sometimes be sources of tension." Avoiding stress-provoking situations and people is something I am working on.

Positive thinking may relieve chronic pain since pain emanates from the brain. Positive thoughts create feelings of well-being causing the brain to increase levels of serotonin and dopamine. Laughing also increases endorphins, signaling safety and calm. Negative thoughts stimulate release of cortisol and adrenaline, the so-called stress hormones. These impact the body by raising heart rate and tensing muscles, with breath becoming shallow. How do we change our brains? Cognitive behavioral therapy can train one to minimize personality traits of perfectionism, catastrophizing, and holding in of emotions which may all contribute to chronic pain. Through repetition we can retrain our brains to change pain-inducing patterns. And if we can epigenetically change our brains, can we interrupt this painful inheritance?

chapter 31

Change Your Mind

Progress is impossible without change, and those who cannot change their minds cannot change anything.
—George Bernard Shaw[47]

A doorstop of a book landed on my porch last week that changed my thinking about migraine. *Migraine in Medicine—a Machine-Generated Overview of Current Research,"* edited by Paolo Martelletti.[48] At over one thousand pages covering abstracts of recent studies throughout the world concerning migraine, it is a goldmine. A.I. meets migraine. I unearth my rusty mining tools and begin sifting for ore. I know that everything is subject to error and even machine generated output is only as good as the input. I consider A.I. to be useful as a stimulus for further exploration.

This is just before my every ninety days round of thirty-one Botox injections, when my brain is at its nadir in intellectual function. The day after Botox, the nerve endings feel frayed and complain, so I peruse the abstracts, take notes, and allow the studies to marinate, while I ice my head on the sofa and dose myself with acetominophen, naratriptan, Nurtec® ODT, (Rimegepant Oral Dissolve Tablet) and Compazine (not all at the same time). Sipping ginger and peppermint teas, I limit myself to three cups of coffee or tea each day. With no appetite, I eat enough for sustenance and supplement my depleted electrolytes, in between napping and reading, while trying to understand what is happening inside my own black box. My cranium has been locked for seventy years and now I am about to glimpse inside of my migraineur's skull.

Are we on the cusp of precision medicine where integrating functional MRI and genetic markers can customize treatment? Prevent migraine?

These are the some of the things I learn:

1. Migraine can drive brain changes, though it is unknown whether this is a disease-causing aspect or an effect of the disease.[49]

2. Migraineurs have alterations in the metabolism of neurotransmitters. This has been found by assays of blood, urine, and cerebrospinal fluid. GABA (gamma-amino-butyric acid), the most widespread inhibitory neurotransmitter in the brain has been implicated in the pathogenesis of migraine. This has been observed in cortical spreading depression which is responsible

for migraine aura and in the activation of the trigeminal vascular system which incites pain.[50]

3. In the 2020 *Journal of Molecular Neuroscience*, "Searching for Predictors of Migraine Chronification: A Pilot Study of 1911AG Polymorphism of TRPV1 Gene in Episodic Versus Chronic Migraine," we are informed that gene expression fluctuates with environmental and endogenous events. **There is a genetic marker which protects an episodic migraineur from progressing to chronic status.**[51]

Alleluia. When can I undergo selective gene-editing to reverse my undeserved life sentence?

4. The most alarming revelation I find during my days of languishing and reading, is in the abstract "A volumetric magnetic resonance imaging study in migraine," published in the *Egyptian Journal of Neurology, Psychiatry, and Neurosurgery* in 2021. The conclusion states "Chronic migraineurs showed significant reduction in grey matter in areas involved with processing of pain, cognition, and multisensory integration versus patients with episodic migraine. This progressive disorder may have long-term impacts on the brain as regards structure and function."[52]

I drop the heavy volume on the floor and my poodle jumps. I need to *change everything* I can to erase the chronic curse. My brain needs a major overhaul, and I am the only one to do it. I live alone and do not want to be enfeebled because of migraine. Shrinkage of my brain is not on my bucket list, and reversing the pain pattern is key to maintaining as many brain cells as possible. Thank goodness I am not much of a drinker, as alcohol consumption has been shown to be deleterious to the lifespan of brain cells.

5. Another stunner was in the abstract "Structural and Functional Brain Changes in Migraine," published in *Pain and Therapy*, 2021. "High frequency of white matter abnormalities, silent infarct-like lesions, and volumetric changes in both white and gray matter have been demonstrated."[53]

My first dizzy thought is to schedule a brain MRI, with and without contrast dye. I am sure my neurologist will order this since it has been many years since my last brain scan, my dizziness has increased, and any change in presentation of migraine should be studied. Perhaps the insurance company will cover it. But then, what if I find that my brain is riddled with nonsense? Resembles Swiss cheese? Is shrunken like a prune? Maybe I do not need to know if I cannot improve the condition. I can only do what I have been doing: living as well as possible, despite chronic migraine. I suppose I could begin interviewing kindly caregivers. My poodle could go for advanced training to be my therapy dog. Second thought: I think I will hold off on getting another brain MRI.

Medical student syndrome (MSS) is a condition that many

medical, nursing, and pharmacy students acquire during their study of disease. Reading of symptoms in medical books may lead to over-interpretation of one's own health state. Cyberchondria is a newer version of this, where internet searches may precipitate undue concern for the disease being researched. If I think I may have brain shrinkage, I may begin to act accordingly. It is a psychosomatic response and is not uncommon. So be informed, but do not search for problems where they may not exist. While I do not believe that ignorance is bliss, I am selective in overturning stones as I seek my own cure.

chapter 32

Reclaim the Brain

Let food be thy medicine and medicine thy food.
—Hippocrates[54]

I am thrilled whenever I talk to a fellow migraineur who has found significant relief. After a course on the campus of Hope College, at the Hope Academy of Senior Professionals, fellow HASPer, Sherry, tells me that her monthly migraine disappeared at menopause. My Aunt Mary Lou told me the same thing. She says she has not endured a single brainstorm since age sixty. Am I a late bloomer at seventy, still searching for my deliverance? I would trade my IRA for a pain-free brain.

I read this past week that some migraineurs report cancellation of migraine with an ophthalmic application of a beta-adrenergic blocker: Timoptic® (timolol 0.5%). This drug is indicated for treatment of glaucoma and is thought to work by reducing production of fluid in the eye which lowers intraocular pressure. By the oral route, beta blockers reduce blood pressure, pulse rate, and induce anti-anxiety effects. Reported side effects with the ophthalmic application include blurred vision, decreased night vision, irritation, and increased risk of cataract formation due to effect on the lens. I am hesitant to use this eye drop because I have some pre-existing ophthalmic conditions. I have taken oral beta-blockers in the past, prescribed as preventative strategy, which resulted in very low blood pressure without obvious improvement in frequency or severity of migraine. However, if a rapid acting dose does not need to pass through the liver before reaching the site of head pain, mitigation may result with less systemic side effects. The ophthalmic dose is thought to enter the nasal cavity through the lacrimal duct. Why not avoid the eyes and cook up a nasal spray?

I dig deeper and find a compounding pharmacy in Kansas City, MO concocting beta-blocker nasal spray, which has been shown to be absorbed as fast as via the intravenous route. Eureka. With an estimated 39 million Americans and one billion people worldwide suffering from migraine, why has not a single pharmaceutical company jumped on this? The beta-blocker itself is cheap, and this class of drug has been used for decades as a preventative treatment for migraine. Of course, this is a new route of administration, and the drug will be used for acute treatment rather than chronic, requiring a new FDA application. Instead of holding my breath awaiting market release of a beta-blocker nasal spray, I request a prescription from my neurologist, and I locate a Michigan compounding pharmacy to mix up a batch for my own trial. If I can snort a treatment and reclaim my brain in fifteen minutes, I am a willing guinea pig. And if a pharmaceutical company launches a study for this application, I will be investing a chunk of my 401K with them. Initial studies with topicals, either ophthalmic or nasal route, have overwhelmingly outperformed placebo without negative effects. Anecdotally, rebound headache has not been observed as with triptans, NSAIDS, and acetaminophen.

An opportunity arises to try out this cool new tool on a day when I am planning to stay home and write. No driving necessary and it is a perfect time to monitor side effects such as low blood pressure. A brainstorm approaches and I spray timolol up my nostrils. I lay down after swallowing two acetominophen 500mg tablets and wait for relief. In thirty minutes, I arise and feel that I am ahead of this storm. Sitting at my desk I smile and revel in the discovery that it seems to be working. I am pain-free until my neighbor down in the valley gasses up his heavy-duty backpack leaf blower and chases a few leaves around his nearly barren yard for a few hours. Up on the sand dune where I live, the window-rattling roar ignites my brain, and the migraine blooms. Despite chilled earplugs and a strong cup of coffee, I slip down my slope into pain. I will try the timolol nasal spray again to see if the relief may be more lasting under quieter circumstances. Though the downside of the treatment is the necessity of traveling to a compounding pharmacy an hour away, paying cash for the prescription, which has a shelf-life of *just one month* for this special preparation. It is probably not a feasible treatment long-term for me, but an option for some. If it were more stable, I would continue to experiment, but the product is about to expire with only one use at about $80. If a pharmaceutical company could make a shelf-stable version of this nasal beta-blocker, it may have a huge market for acute brainstorms.

With so many types of migraine, is it any wonder that we have difficulty selecting the best treatment? Here are a few subtypes of migraine I have discovered in the literature over many decades of personal research:

1. Migraine with aura: which provides a warning that allows the victim to line up the artillery (medications). An aura may have provided inspiration for Lewis Carroll's "Adventures of Alice in Wonderland." Blind spots, lines, zig-zag-like lightning, flashing and flickering lights, temporary loss of vision, dizziness, and more presage the brainstorm. White rabbit hallucinations are optional.

2. Chronic migraine: occurs on fifteen or more days per month for at least three months.

3. Migraine with brainstem aura may cause tinnitus, double vision, syncope, changes in eyesight in both eyes, tingling of arms and legs, slurring of speech as if having a stroke. This type occurs in about 10% of migraineurs.

4. Retinal or Ocular migraine: causes transient scotoma, missing visual areas in one eye.

5. Vestibular migraine: dizzy type, not necessarily blonde.

6. Abdominal migraine: my niece experienced this before the onset of puberty with severe nausea and vomiting. It was debilitating at the time, though she outgrew it.

7. Hemiplegic migraine: causes paralysis on one side of the body, usually an arm or leg.

8. Menstrual migraine: usually appears with other premenstrual symptoms. Can also show up mid-cycle with ovulation. Estrogen fluctuations are known migraine triggers. This is why migraine may disappear during pregnancy and after menopause.

9. Migraine without aura: the most common type. The bad news is that these patients may not recognize the approach of a migraine and wait too long to address it. The migraine gallops out of control, medication overuse may ensue, and chronic migraine may develop. But the good news is that migraine patients without aura do not have a higher incidence of stroke, as those with aura do. This is my type, and I am grateful for a lower incidence of stroke. (My gratitude for the day.)

chapter 33

How to Help a Migraineur

Don't sweat the petty things and don't pet the sweaty things.
—George Carlin[55]

One of the most frequent questions I get from people who have not experienced migraine is, what causes your headaches? Answer: If I could find the cause and correct it, do you think I would be suffering for the past fifty-eight years? Or, according to the *Journal of Neurology, Psychiatry and Brain Research*, Volume 31, February 2019, page 20, "Exact etiology of migraine, uncertain, none of the hitherto postulated mechanisms sufficiently explain the pathogenesis of migraine."[56]

I do not answer this way. Most often I say: "I do not know." Or if they press for an answer, I say: "weather." This is truthful. It is one of my triggers. Some non-migraineurs are befuddled when the sun shines and I hide indoors, mired in migraine while they head to the beach. "Isn't it a lovely day?" Feck, no. Not audibly. Or on 'soft' days (as they say in Ireland), when I do not have a migraine, and I lace up my boots for a hike between raindrops, they shake their heads, refusing to join me. Do they sport Jello-flesh? Are they afraid of melting? Probably not, but they have more options for hiking, biking, kayaking, and carefree living since they are not migraineurs. These lucky ducks can plan days and weeks ahead for their hikes, whereas I tend to seize any day before it seizes me.

I believe that a particular load of triggers will push a susceptible individual from wellness into brainstorm. Sometimes my brainstorm feels like I am taking a cold shower under Niagara Falls. The pressure is so intense that my entire body throbs. Affecting about thirty-nine million Americans, the best guesses for contributing factors of chronic migraine are genetics, environmental, serotonin levels, blood glucose levels, and electrical activity in the brain. I think it is all the above.

I hear from well-meaning friends who "have heard of a miracle cure on TV that you must try. It's called Excedrin Migraine®." Or their cousin banished her migraine by switching to a vegan, no-gluten diet. Or a keto diet. Or had a Daith piercing of the inner cartilage fold of the ear. Or . . .

Some researchers are studying ketogenesis for migraineurs since it has been a therapeutic tool for epilepsy since 1920. And a lot of epilepsy drugs are used off-label for migraine since they are both brain disorders. There is an involved scientific explanation of why keto may be helpful, and it boils down to something regarding the Krebs cycle. *Una piccola* Italian study consisted of a pair of young, obese twins, placed on a Keto Diet for weight loss. Both had a remarkable decrease in migraine frequency after three days (forgoing pasta and pizza). However, I am not sold on a high fat, ketogenic diet since it has been shown to increase cardiovascular disease. If I had an optimal blood lipids profile or was thirty years old, I would experiment with ketogenesis. However, I do appreciate the concern of friends. I have tried most every drug and diet and if it was helpful, I would adhere to it.

What would be helpful to a migraineur?

Can I walk your dog? Get your mail? Make soup or toast or tea? Pick up a prescription? Load an icepack? Grab groceries? Shovel the driveway? Enlist an exorcist? Mostly, a migraineur needs a quiet place to ride out the current episode. Darkness, solitude, warm hands and toes, and a cold head ease my migraine.

And how do you know when a brainstorm is on your loved one's doorstep? Many patients have prodromes, warnings, that sneak up and presage an attack. This may occur days to hours before the actual event. I find difficulty in concentration, slowed mental processing, fatigue, emotional changes, visual aberrations, food cravings, and sometimes extra yawning or sneezing, but I have allergies too. Language slips out my door just before a migraine visits, memory clouds, and my equilibrium shifts to vertigo mode. If I am dizzy, crabby, and cannot remember your name, a brainstorm approaches. And when it lands, use your indoor voice, please.

Migraineurs will experience pain, cognitive dysfunction, nausea, photophobia (sensitive eyes), and phonophobia (sensitive hearing). My family and friends say it is easier to beat me at Scrabble™ when I am under a brainstorm since my vocabulary is limited. Does this collateral bonus outweigh my diminished self? I am here to please you. Can you please walk my poodle?

chapter 34

NAPPING 101

Throw me to the wolves and I will return
leading the pack.
—Seneca[57]

After I get thirty minutes of shut eye.
—Susan P. Ryan

While I was growing up, napping was for babies and sick people. I did not nap and found it hard to rest even when I felt slammed by a brainstorm. I worked through whatever ailment I had, including migraine, since there was always work to do or fun to pursue. I considered napping as a sign of weakness. I got by on less than eight hours of sleep since I was a night owl and always had a job awaiting me in the morning. When my migraine evolved from episodic to chronic, i.e., fifteen or more days per month for three months or more, I still had a tough time resting. On the days I was without pain, I pushed myself harder than ever, trying to reclaim time lost to migraine. I have learned that it is not possible to catch up on sleep, rest, or work. We will always have a deficit. But, in recent years I have found that a thirty-minute power nap can do wonders for focus and energy level. Though I love my coffee and tea, caffeine is not always the best answer. Napping is my new muse. I do not nap every day, but whenever I am home and fading in the afternoon, I may collapse on the sofa, floor, or bed to recharge my batteries. If my after-lunch coffee does not lift me enough, I lay down with my poodle puppy for thirty minutes and find that this is what my body needs at this time. If I cannot sleep, I meditate, pray, and lower my level of concern. If I pay attention to my body's cues and ease up on the accelerator, I am ultimately more productive.

During my career in the medical field, napping was not a luxury I could afford, nor could I slow myself down enough to sleep during daylight hours, despite migraine. This constant drive may have pushed me into the chronic migraine category. And now I am trying to reverse this trend. Some months, I have less than fifteen headache days. And whenever I have a week without a single headache, I am thrilled and believe that I am on the path to healing my brain. It took a long time to get to this point, and I expect that a cure will be gradual. I work on it every day while doing my utmost to sleep better at night. There is no better medicine than sleep.

chapter 35

SMILE AWHILE

It's not what happens to you, but how you react to it that matters.[58]
—Epictetus

Sometimes my life sucks, but if I keep moving, the clouds vaporize, my brainstorm lifts off, and the good life returns. I often feel so well that I imagine that the migraine curse is just a bad dream. I am a poseur. It cannot be all that bad. Does amnesia supplant pain? After undergoing childbirth, does every woman say: "never again?" We would all lack siblings. Endorphins erase the memory of pain and smiling has been shown to increase endorphin production. Distraction of any sort is helpful. I am not a television watcher, but occasionally I may get lost in a film that removes me from my state of pain as I wander about a distant realm as an observer. Or into a novel as a bystander to someone else's life.

This morning, I awake before sunrise feeling well and pain free, unusual for me this past year, and I savor this surge of well-being for a few moments. When I arise, a dizziness descends, nausea ensues, and I barely get down my breakfast of oatmeal with blueberries and walnuts. I am no longer headed in the right direction. I mix up a glass of electrolytes, swallow a triptan and two extra strength acetaminophen. After breakfast I drink two cups of pour-over coffee. Fully medicated, I decide to reduce a stack of *Wall Street Journals* from the past week, catching up on the world in between naps on the sofa with an icepack on my head. I could call it a wasted day but let me say "it is a relaxing Sunday," dictated by this migraine brain. It is not my choice to change plans, but my dizzy brain cancels church, grocery shopping, and a sunny hike on this fine winter day. I can wallow in misery, or I can do what is best for me at this time: resting. I let go of my schedule, I ride out the brainstorm, and seven hours later the vertigo dissipates. I am grateful that the pain never reaches more than five on a scale of ten, though I spend the day inside a fuzzy tunnel. My eyes close whenever the sun peeks through the March clouds, revealing a vivid blue I have not seen since last year. I am too dizzy to search for sunglasses, so I melt into the sofa and occasionally toss a soggy tennis ball to my young Spoo (standard poodle). Vinny is learning patience, and he tries to comfort me, pressing his moist, stuffing-shedding lamb under my head. I am charmed by his empathy and ability to locate the source of my pain.

I prepare a simple supper of roasted vegetables and poached eggs while looking forward to a better day tomorrow. Warm and safe, I live in a comfortable home with a loving puppy, a fuzzy gentleman-in-training. Without the brainstorms, I may not be as appreciative of what I have, though I know that I can accomplish more while pain-free. Someone once said I was "a human-doing rather than a human-being." Migraine is slowing me down for some reason. Making me more human. Smile.

It took four decades for my episodic migraine to cross over into chronic territory. I am trying my best to unwind this troubled mind, to reset its super-sensitivity to something less reactive, and to enjoy a less-burdened decade or two.

I emerge from the whirling fog in time for bed, looking forward to Monday morning. Smile.

Reclaim the brain. I try to squeeze as much life as possible out of each day. Some days it may be an ounce or less, but on days without migraine I fill a reservoir with gratitude. And whenever I enjoy a week of migraine-free days, I tend to forget how all-encompassing they are. In the words of Tadej Pogacar, 2024 winner of the Tour de France, "I erase my memories if they are bad. I'm like a goldfish." And like a goldfish, I hop on my bike and pedal. I never look behind me and never expect to be overtaken by a faster fish.

chapter 36

Twenty-First Century Headache

Insanity is doing the same thing over and over and expecting different results.
—Albert Einstein[59]

Though migraine is one of the top causes of disability throughout the world, most sufferers self-treat rather than seek out specialized medical advice. Digital technology confers autodidactic medical degrees on the masses without tuition expense and long years of study. With so many websites offering advice for migraineurs, it is easy to feel that proffered prescriptions are specific to our needs. Patients are likely to pop Excedrin Migraine since it is so well-marketed and labelled as a "migraine" treatment. It is inexpensive, contains aspirin, acetaminophen, and caffeine, all well-known ingredients that may alleviate one's head pain. In fact, this combination will work for many sufferers, for a time. Though if taken more than three days in a week or ten days in a month, this type of drug may cause more headaches. This condition is called MOH (medication overuse headache). There are prescription drugs that will also cause MOH if used too often. I was a too-frequent user of triptans for my too-frequent migraine days since this remedy alone stopped the pain when nothing else lifted the burden. When my brainstorms would not depart for more than a day, I was hospitalized seven days for detox. I describe this in chapter thirteen: Impatient Inpatient. My headaches morphed from the episodic category into chronic, considered by the medical establishment to be fifteen or more migraine days per month for at least three months. This is not trivial. It continues over a decade later.

My advice to avoid becoming a chronic migraineur:

- Find a neurologist who specializes in migraine. Look online and/or ask your primary care provider for a referral. There is a paucity of headache specialists, but they are key to better management of migraine. If you can prevent the frequency from increasing to chronic level, your quality of life will be vastly improved.

- If doing research online, look at medical sites such as Mayo Clinic, Johns Hopkins, Universities with medical schools, etc. You may find information that will be useful in discussing your migraine with your physician.

- Chart headache days on a calendar, noting medications used, relief obtained, severity of pain on a scale of 1-5 or 1-10. This record will be helpful for your treatment.

- If you have more than a monthly migraine, do not pass go, do not stop at Urgent Care, but seek out your personal specialist. Find one who listens to you, rather than looking at you, drugging you, and billing you. You are not generic. Your care should be specific.

- Consult with a behavioral therapist to learn coping skills to reduce stress, a major trigger.

- Be sure to weigh the benefits of medications and supplements against their side effects. Less is more when taking drugs. **Avoid medication overuse headaches.**

- I believe that the best treatment involves sound sleep on a regular schedule with quality more important than quantity.

- Consume a healthy diet without preservatives and additives, avoiding alcohol and anything neurotoxic. If uncertain about what is a healthy diet, visit a nutritionist.

- Maintain good hydration in all seasons. Carry water with you, preferably in a reusable container, rather than plastic.

- Enjoy daily moderate exercise as part of your routine.

- Identify and avoid your triggers.

If you treat your episodic migraine eruptions adequately, you may be able to prevent chronic migraine, something I have been trying to escape for far too long. Studies show that about 2.5% of episodic migraineurs convert each year to chronic. Converting back to episodic is possible, but I have not yet turned my tide. I am searching for the key to remodel my over-reactive brain. Though we do not have any migraine cures yet, many migraine-specific drugs have been introduced in the last few years. Be informed and involved in your health. No one is going to cure you, but you can improve your quality of life.

End of lecture.

chapter 37

COGNITIVE IMPACTS

Inspiration arrives as a packet of material to be delivered.
— John Updike[60]

Unfortunately, that package is undeliverable during brainstorm.
—Susan P. Ryan

Migraineurs may experience significant memory deficits during a brainstorm compared to other types of headaches. Isn't that special, though I am grateful that my headaches are rarely as painful as they once were, when it felt like an icepick piercing my left eye socket. This relief may be due to the newer treatments of Botox to numb the forehead and neck muscles and dampen input to corresponding cranial nerves. CGRP inhibitors may add to this effect of moderating brain pain. However, nausea, dizziness, and loss of words are still debilitating. I look like a fully functioning adult, sporting a fake smile, until someone asks me, "What is her name?" or "What are you doing?" And I cannot answer coherently. Why is my brain still fuzzy when the pain has been downsized?

Chronic pain and its accessories seep into each cell of one's being. Sometimes it is just background noise, with twinges that are mildly annoying. Other times it flares like wildfire and erases the rest of the world. Normally an agile communicator, during a brainstorm I am unable to hold up my side of a conversation, searching for words and coming up with nonsense, as if I am having a stroke. It is a brain attack, and the verbal part of my brain is affected. According to University of California at San Francisco Speech and Language Weill Institute of Neurosciences, "Broca's area, located in the left hemisphere, is associated with speech production and articulation. Our ability to articulate ideas, as well as use words accurately in spoken and written language, has been attributed to this crucial area." [61]

My Broca is broken but my comprehension seems intact when I am limited in my ability to say the correct words. Fortunately, my Wernicke's area is not (yet) involved. Impairment of this area causes one to speak in a word salad that the speaker feels is correct but cannot be understood by others. While I am grateful for this blessing, my motor skills are diminished as I deal with dizziness, holding onto walls and furniture whenever I am upright. I feel clumsy and stagger as if drunk.

When the brainstorm departs, it leaves behind its shadow. Within the shadow lie unspoken or misspoken words, a memory of loss, and a glimpse of eternity. This respite from pain inspires

Cognitive Impacts

me to press on, to seize my pain-free days and squeeze more life out of each one. I am grateful for each precious moment devoid of migraine, and I continue to search for my cure.

chapter 38

PATIENTS ARE NOT GENERIC

I give you bitter pills in sugar coating. The pills are harmless; the poison is in the sugar.
—Stanislaw Jerzey Lec [62]

Before you refill another prescription, you may want to pick up a copy of *Bottle of Lies: The Inside Story of the Generic Drug Boom* by investigative journalist Katherine Eban.[63] Americans, perhaps, vocally leading a worldwide outcry, are clamoring for lower drug prices and our government is pressuring the FDA to approve generic drugs faster to fulfill this need. However, the FDA is not able to inspect each offshore manufacturing plant with surprise visits as happens in the U.S. This book is an exposé of the lack of oversight of safe manufacturing standards in countries where most of our generics are made. The active pharmaceutical agents used in manufacture of drugs are produced in the following locations: 13% in the U.S., 28% in India, 17% in China, 30% in Europe, 4% non-US Americas, 8% other Asia. This raw material is used in manufacturing the final dose forms which are produced in the following countries: 40% US, 4% non-U.S. Americas, 19% Europe, 23% India, 8% China, 6% other Asia. This information is taken from the article "We Still Don't Know Who Makes This Drug" by Rena M. Conti, Ernst R. Berndt, Neriman Beste Kaygisiz, Yashna Shivdasani, February 7, 2020. *Health Affairs Forefront.*

A few quotes from this article caused me to lose sleep:

1. "The time to worry is now: The coronavirus in China could threaten pharma's ingredient sourcing." Most of our eggs are in this basket, and with the current posturing of the Chinese Communist Party against the west, we should all be concerned about "the vulnerability of America's pharmaceutical supply chain."

2. "U.S. demand for 'off-patent' generic drugs has grown substantially in the last few decades; today more than 90 percent of retail pharmaceutical drug prescriptions in the U.S. are dispensed as generics."

3. "In the past two decades the supply of largely generic prescription drugs to the U.S. market has been repeatedly rocked by shortages. A shortage in Vincristine is the latest one to wreak havoc in the care of pediatric cancer."

4. "Very serious lapses in the quality of manufacturing Valsartan blood pressure medication—-recall for cancer risk with Valsartan, Losartan, a commonly used blood pressure lowering drug, and related 'sartan' products have also been revealed."[64]

There is much more to explore, and a deeper dive is likely to induce a brain attack due to the alarming lack of quality control in this vital industry. When I first started to delve into generic drugs and the role of the FDA, what I read nearly set my hair on fire. It is beyond the scope of this book and warrants further research. But back to my own recent experience with a "generic equivalent." For over a decade I have been taking without any adverse effect, a hormone, progesterone, as part of a regimen to level out hormonal fluctuations, implicated in migraine, as well as prevention of further bone loss after too many rounds of steroids to break up unrelenting migraine. Insurance companies practice medicine by switching patients from brand name drugs to generics to save costs. Sometimes a generic substitute is a seamless move, but during reformulations, chemical changes are implemented by generic manufacturers to avoid patent infringement. And despite these alterations, this new drug is considered a "generic equivalent." However, the medication may not react the same way as the original drug formulation. And in a haste to get generic drugs to market before competitors, corners are often cut, with quality compromised according to a generic company's whistleblower in Eban's book.

When my pharmacy filled my prescription about three years ago with an Indian pharmaceutical company's "generic equivalent" progesterone, I experienced postmenopausal vaginal bleeding, an alarming side effect, which often results in biopsy or surgery to rule out cancer. Alarmed, I called the pharmacy and was told "generic formulations are all different, but the active ingredients are the same." With my background in pharmacy, I understand that this side effect was caused by an inaccurate quantity of active ingredient, not pharmaceutical fillers. I tried a few refills with different lots of this product since this is what the pharmacy offered to me. Each batch of this company's progesterone caused the same alarming issue. This manufacturer was the "preferred" company for this pharmacy chain's warehouse. I filed two separate complaints with the FDA, offered to send my unused meds for Q.A. testing, **but never received a response**. It is alarming that the FDA has so little regard for patients. Do they not work for U.S. taxpayers?

Whenever I pick up prescriptions, I now ask for the country of origin and request other options when the response is either India or China. Pharmacy chain stores are limited to certain manufacturers, dictated by what their warehouses stock, all chosen on basis of cost. When I sold heart valves, a purchasing agent told me that my product was more expensive than my competitor's. I asked him, "If your wife or child required a heart valve replacement, would you select the cheapest valve or the valve with the best long term-term clinical performance?"

First do no harm.

In Eban's book, a particular drug was found to *vary from pill to pill by 45 percent in quantity of active ingredient*. This can be a matter of life and death for certain medications. The author writes of dire consequences for patients who depend on anti-rejection drugs following organ transplantation. Patients died from organ rejection after taking generic drugs which were found to contain inadequate dosages. Cheaper, but deadly in their ineffectiveness. Some drugs are designed to dispense a gradual amount of active ingredient over time, but with poor formulation, the entire dose is rapidly absorbed with disastrous effects. Cardiac drugs, chemotherapeutics, anti-epileptics, antihypertensives, diabetes management drugs, and injectables are all high on the list of potential for serious harm if the formulated generics are not *safe and effective*.

We migraineurs take many drugs, some with an indication for migraine and others used "off-label." And we will receive generic drugs after patents expire. We may be subjected to unexpected new side effects as well as lack of effectiveness. If the FDA cannot guarantee that our imported generic drugs are safe and effective and perform like the brand name drugs they replace, we should not purchase them from abroad. They should be manufactured in the U.S. and tested for safety and effectiveness. All generics are not equivalent. If your results vary with different manufacturers' generic versions of the same drug, talk to your doctor and pharmacist. A generic drug should be equivalent, but is it?

chapter 39

Monoclonal Antibodies 2.0

Lend yourself to others but give yourself to yourself.
—Michel de Montaigne [65]

While poking me with darts of poison, my current neurologist says, "I am not happy with the frequency of your migraine. You need to try some other preventative meds. Do you still want to continue with Botox?"

"Yes, though it does not diminish the frequency, my pain level is reduced. I am just overwhelmed by cognitive dysfunction, dizziness, and inability to articulate."

"Let's try nerve blocks in between the rounds of Botox and add Qulipta® (atogepant), an oral CGRP inhibitor that you will take every day. Discontinue the monthly Emgality injections, and no more Nurtec as your abortive med."

After two rounds of jarring nerve blocks at the base of my skull and into the eyebrows, I experience no reduction in pain other than the hour or so immediately after the treatment while I sit in my car, experiencing scalp numbness and a floaty feeling which keeps me parked. I unpack lunch, nibble a peanut butter and peach jam sandwich on cherry walnut sourdough bread, and sip hot coffee, grateful that I had planned to have emergency provisions on hand. I have attended more than a few rodeos. Closing my eyes, I lean my swollen noggin against the headrest and try to savor the temporary absence, or perhaps it is an apathy of pain. I have migraine, but it feels more distant than its usual undeniable manifestation. I wait, breathe deeply, and wonder when I may be fit to drive home or optimistically to make a grocery stop. After a few more rounds, I determine that the nerve blocks do not make a difference in the frequency of my migraine, so we move on to the newest med.

The pharmacy calls to inform me that a month supply of Qulipta 60mg will be $1,200. "It's non-formulary, but we can ask your doctor to submit a prior authorization." An hour later the pharmacy calls with news. It is December and I have racked up enough prescription costs for the calendar year to put me in "the catastrophic category," qualifying for a $55 co-pay. Hot dog! This reminds me of the frequent flyer points I racked up during my career of business travel. I was sometimes upgraded to a business class seat. Of course, the airlines never used the word "catastrophic" in their marketing. After two months of this special price, my February co-pay increases to $500 per month for 30 tablets. If there were no side effects and a slight decrease in frequency, I would pay without complaint. But I experience severe constipation despite lots of fruit, fiber, fluids, and laxatives. January 2024, *twenty-one migraine days*, a new personal record in this decade. The neurologist says it may take up to three months to see improvement, so we stay on this course for a few more weeks. My optimism wanes and I become more devout with my prayers. I have always thought that it is selfish to pray for one's own health while so many others are suffering with worse maladies, but I now believe that it may be time to change that thinking. Help me also, Lord.

February, *eighteen migraine days* in this short month with side effects interrupting my sleep. A few days short of the 90-day prescribed trial, I drop this expensive experiment, give myself an injection of Emgality, stored in my refrigerator, and pick up a refill of Nurtec 75mg, #8 tablets for $375. This is my backup for when I have used my maximum of three doses of naratriptan in a week. The price per pill of Nurtec should be enough to incite a placebo effect, but it does not seem any better than no drug. On my next visit with the neurologist in four weeks, I plan to ask about switching to Frova, which has the longest half-life of all triptans. I am running out of options. A cooling gel strip (with camphor as the active ingredient), plastered on my forehead seems to provide a bit of relief. It is at least a useful distraction. I need to get back to my former life before chronicity becomes irreversible.

chapter 40

Time—Healer or Thief?

I don't so much fear death as I do wasting life.
—Oliver Sacks.[66]

Our clocks are wound and running, and from this we cannot escape. Beyond good health, time is my next most valuable consideration. I feel like I am always trying to catch up, to recover time after migraine has stolen my day(s). I crank into hyperdrive once the fog lifts, and I often overwork myself into another brainstorm. Moderation is a foreign language I am trying to learn. Zen is my goal. Upon googling a useful definition, I land on this:

> *Zen is the Japanese pronunciation of a Chinese word, ch'an, which comes from a Sanskrit root meaning thought, absorption, or meditation. And meditation is at the heart of Zen along with an emphasis on self-control and insight.*

Insight. That is a key word for me. I google further and find:

> *Eight Zen-Living Tips That Can Change Your Life:*
> 1. *Keep only what is necessary. Zen living means removing items that are not necessary to your life.*
> 2. *Allow space.*
> 3. *Adopt a simple way of living.*
> 4. *Live mindfully.*
> 5. *Don't multitask.*
> 6. *Do less.*
> 7. *Meditate.*
> 8. *Be grateful.*[67]

I will not purge my closets and bookshelves today, but I will begin to declutter my space as soon as the present brainstorm passes. Multitasking has been my way of life and should be beaten (or eased) into submission. Shall I toss out my smarter than me iPhone or use it only at certain times of the day? It is an intrusion which scrambles my attention. But how much less can I do when I am shackled to my sofa for days each week? Deep breath. On fair days I will focus on a few priorities.

I make a point of being grateful each morning when I open my eyes. A decent night's sleep incites my utmost gratitude. Thank you, Lord, I intone as I stretch my limbs and vow to savor each pain-free minute of this day. My family buried another sweet aunt this weekend and I find myself subtracting my age from hers, calculating my remaining time. I am savoring the heck out of this 39-degree May 1st, with rain splattering my windows and the lake roaring at the end of the street. I am alive and the storm remains outside my head. I am blessed and I will do my best to perpetuate this blessing by being mindful. Time is healing my head. I am hopeful that this cure is lasting.

chapter 41

CHRONIC/IRONIC

Embrace the suck.[68]
—A U.S. Marine shared this motto with me.

Copy.
—Susan P. Ryan

After another slide to the dark side, that is, more than fifteen days per month with migraine, I sign up for an OLLI (Oschner Lifelong Learning Institute) course,[69] watching it via Zoom on a snowy January day. The topic is Chronic Pain, and the presenter is Daniel Clauw, M.D., Professor of Anesthesiology, Internal Medicine, Rheumatology, and Psychiatry at the University of Michigan. He is director of the Chronic Pain and Fatigue Research Center. At the conclusion of his two-hour lecture, I am about to call for an appointment to meet this genius, when he informs the audience that he no longer sees patients in his office but does research full-time and dishes out advice to colleagues who have gotten away from prescribing opioids post-operatively. Rats. But I will share some of the notes I took during his presentation.

Clauw talks about a "volume control setting" in the brain which he explains is the issue behind chronic pain. To alleviate pain, the setting needs to be dialed down. Drugs for depression, such as Cymbalta® (duloxetine), a selective serotonin and norepinephrine reuptake inhibitor are commonly prescribed as a method to "dial down the pain setting." This drug works well for fibromyalgia, and it sounds like a good idea for some chronic migraineurs, but the side effects have not been compatible with my physiology.

Clauw studies the endocannabinoid system where the body's own pain killer is produced. This system was unknown when I attended pharmacy school in the 70s, though reefer madness infected the campus, with a skunky fog hanging over the Diag each April 1 during Hash Bash. Just walking to class on central campus gave students a "contact high." Doc says that CBD is a safe and effective anti-inflammatory. I tried it for several months, scoring a "high quality" formulation in Ann Arbor with no noticeable effect on my migraine frequency, though it may help some sufferers. Since there are no cannabinoid receptors in the brainstem, patients do not die from cannabis overdose, though many end up in the ER with hyperemesis. (Kind of like some patients in the throes of migraine.) When I experimented with cannabis, I felt extremely nauseous, though maybe it was a bad batch of peanuts. The THC-laced peanut butter was not labelled with the place of origin and processing, concentration of active ingredients, nor the list of other ingredients, just a recommended dosage of *1/8th teaspoonful on a cracker at the onset of pain.* I spoke with a compounding pharmacist recently, who says that his pharmacy does not manufacture gummies or use viscous carriers, since it is difficult to insure accurate doses. The margin for error should be less than 2 percent but may be much higher due to inconsistency in mixing of thick ingredients like peanut butter. After my reaction of tachycardia, nausea, vomiting, and room-spinning dizziness, I toss out this experiment. I likely scooped up a stronger than expected dose of THC, which put me over the edge of safety and effectiveness.

Clauw recommends, "Start with CBD alone, then add a low dose of THC if needed. This should not make one "high" if the CBD is greater in concentration than the THC." I have been taking the CBD capsules for a few months before I ingest the THC peanut butter during a painful brainstorm. Is the ratio of CBD:THC inverted? Until I see real quality control, accurate labeling of strength, prescribing advice from pharmacists and/or physicians, prospective randomized studies, showing a 50% or greater reduction in the number of migraines without ugly side effects, I am not retreading the cannabis path.

According to Clauw, there are other ways to decrease the "volume control setting" to reduce pain:

Deep sleep and enough sleep. I am doing everything I can to sleep better.

Be physically active. This raises serotonin and norepinephrine without side effects.

YES!

Caloric restriction may decrease pain. Low blood sugar triggers migraine for me, so I am working on smaller portions rather than intermittent fasting.

Low glutamate diet. (no MSG, artificial sweeteners)

Gluten-free diet may decrease pain. I try this for six weeks without any change in migraine frequency. And I test negative for gluten sensitivity with a blood test and colon biopsy. I am currently trying another round of no gluten for 90 days and will add back small amounts next month. Some sources decry gluten as "inflammatory," but it may be related to dose.

Using functional MRI, non-drug treatments are shown to be effective without side effects.

The brain shrinks with chronic pain. This neuroplasticity may be a mechanism to decrease pain since all pain arises in the brain. This remodeling of the nervous system changes both the size and shape of the brain.

This is chilling to me. Not wanting to lose any more brain cells than necessary, I am doing everything I can to avoid daily pain. This finding is reason enough to get me outside every single day for a walk. Even with a pounding, resounding, dizzying migraine, just a bit of a walk. With sunglasses and a hat. The poodle appreciates this.

chapter 42

PLATELETS—PERHAPS

It is necessary to keep one's compass in one's eyes and not in the hand, for the hands execute, but the eye judges.
—Michelangelo[70]

A year ago, my primary care/sports medicine physician injected my arthritic knee joints with PRP, platelet rich plasma, obtained by centrifuging my blood and taking off the resultant golden-colored, platelet-rich top layer of plasma, and injecting this into both knees. Doc says that this treatment "works like fertilizer on the cartilage." On MRI my knee cartilage appears a bit ragged and worn from a life of dare-devilry and high heel hiking around hospitals. But at least I have some knee cartilage remaining for this experiment in rejuvenation. I also tore soft tissues attached to the knee during a full contact gardening misadventure in my sloped backyard this past spring. I limped around for weeks on crutches and finally felt strong enough for a power-boost of healing platelets.

Doc uses an ultrasound to identify landmarks and the best sites for injection. It is not comfortable, but tolerable. My sister Patti attends this appointment with me, curious, since she is facing knee replacements. Doc explains, "for the treatment to work, you must have adequate cartilage." Poor Patti's knees are "bone on bone" with no functional cushion to seed for possible regrowth. Patti drives me home after the procedure since my right knee is stiff and swollen. After the swelling subsides in several weeks, I notice a reduction in knee pain. It is worth the out-of-pocket cost for bilateral injections. ($500 for one knee, $800 for both.) When gardening season returns in the spring, I may consider another round of cartilage fertilizer if needed.

Note: After several months of healing following the knee injections, I am calling this treatment a success. The swelling is noticeably less, the pain is minimal, if I avoid kneeling, tough for a Catholic. And I am now able to bicycle and hike without knee pain. Yippie! Only my roses are being fertilized this year.

PRP has been helping patients since the 1970s, initially to treat low platelet counts. During the 1980s, PRP was used in cardiovascular surgery due to its anti-inflammatory and cell growth propensities. In the 1990s, sports medicine initiated PRP use for muscle and joint injuries in professional athletes. In 2010, dermatologists began subcutaneous injections of PRP for tissue reproduction, wound healing, and to reverse hair loss. PRP can improve burn scars, post-surgical scars, and acne scarring. Though PRP is one of the most promising therapeutic treatments in regenerative medicine, it is cash-only, since it is not covered by insurance. Though it is much less expensive than hospitalization and recovery from knee replacement surgery, insurance companies will not cover PRP treatment. Big Pharma controls medicine, and since there is nothing to patent, it cannot find a way to make money off our body's own healing potential. Is there collusion between drug companies and insurance companies?

To offer PRP treatment, a physician's office must invest in a centrifuge and an ultrasound, but these are not exotic equipment. The per patient cost is dramatically less than replacement knees and rehabilitation. Do lobbyists, politicians, and insurance companies run the health care industry? No need to answer. It seems that the bigger the business, of less importance is the actual customer, the patient. Just wait until we have "Medicare for all." American health care will then be rationed à la Canada and Europe.

With significant improvement in my knees, I wonder: Is there a way to use PRP to minimize my raging brainstorm? One of my friends, who has been a nurse for forty years, suggests that I visit friends of hers who have started a clinic for TruDOSE™ (PRP IV) Therapy in the Louisville area. Sandi has undergone a treatment and says she feels better, good enough to win three recent road-running races in her over 70 age group. And she says her brain fog has diminished. I research online and the only so-called "migraine treatments" I can find using PRP are with local multiple injections. This reportedly also grows hair, so I will keep it in mind in case alopecia appears. I currently endure 31 stunning Botox injections in my tender head and neck every 90 days, resulting in a slight decrease in sensitivity, following a week of needle-induced brainstorm, but I have not realized a reduced frequency of migraine. How can local injections in my head affect the source of my pain, the brain, protected by its bony fortress? The dose needs to be systemic to reach the brain. It must cross the blood-brain barrier. And yes, platelets are tiny and can reach this intended target through the bloodstream.

It is time for March Madness™ [71] in the Midwest, and lured by an earlier spring, the poodle and I load the Honda Odyssey minivan and head six hours south to my old Kentucky hometown, where I lived for 22 years, and where I now open my wallet and offer my pained brain as a human sacrifice to modern medicine. It is about 4 pm on Saturday when we climb the stairs to the new clinic in an old building in a small town outside of Louisville. This rehabbed loft smells of fresh paint and hope. Sitting in a recliner beside my friend Sandi, RN, chatting with two additional registered nurses who are friends with Sandi, I feel relaxed and ready for this new cure. Sandi offers to start my IV since she is arguably the most experienced venipuncturist in the room. I remember years ago when she was waking up in the recovery room, following a long surgery. I was visiting this hospital on business and decided to check on her. Sandi was not pleased with her recovery room nurse who was unable to access her vein for a blood draw after several attempts. Sandi told him, "Just line me up and I'll do the job." Recovering from anesthesia and lying flat in bed, Sandi got the job done on first try. Of course, I agree to bare my arm to Sandi. She says she had been eyeing my veins earlier in the day, saying "piece of cake." Her technique was so smooth that I did not feel a thing and could not find a puncture mark when I removed the pressure bandage before bedtime.

180ml of my blood is withdrawn in three large syringes. This is about six ounces, quite a bit more than was used in the knee PRP injections. An initial finger stick blood test shows my platelet concentration per ml. This information is used to calculate the volume of blood necessary for a therapeutic dose of platelets which in my case is 2.20 billion platelets, based on AI, using data from prior patients. My blood is centrifuged twice, and the top layer of the platelet rich plasma is pushed into my vein via a 10ml syringe through the IV setup. A calm envelops me as the turbo charged platelets tumble through my veins. I am told to relax for a few days and let the PRP do its work. I am told it is regenerative, anti-inflammatory, and healing for whatever needs healing. Body, heal thyself. I write a check for $1,250 for this potential cure. Driving back to Sandi's home through the lush, green horse farm countryside, I layer a few healing prayers onto this latest treatment.

We are both exhausted and head to our bedrooms with our respective canines after a late, light supper. Sandi took first-place running in a seven-mile road race that morning and I played human guinea pig a few hours earlier. Sleeping soundly until 3 am, I sit up in bed. I am now alert as if it is daybreak, and I am enveloped in an endorphin buzz. I feel as if I have just completed a century, a 100-mile bicycle ride in the rolling bluegrass of Kentucky, something I had done in the past, and I am giddy with this sensation. Lying awake for about an hour, I wonder how long this high will last. The next morning, I pack up the minivan still feeling pretty darn good. It is time to head home after a relaxing six-day vacation of visiting old friends. Driving through Indiana,

I stop every two hours for coffee and expand my lungs with fresh air. Why am I so sleepy?

Back home beside Lake Michigan, as the barometric pressure swells and dips, my brain reverberates, and I am afflicted with migraine on four days during the first week post TruDOSE treatment. But in between the brainstorms, I feel better than usual. My lower back pain due to spinal stenosis is nearly gone, and my usual brain fog stays away for eleven blissful days. Is the treatment worth $1,250? I would say YES, though I do not expect an instant cure for a decades-long affliction which has remodeled my brain, with pain as its current default mode. I will give it time and a few more doses since I see no better options. My middle name is Patricia, not Patience. But while feeling like Wonder Woman, or someone without chronic brainstorm, I imagine that I will undergo another treatment in a few months. Meanwhile, I remain optimistic, enjoying a Mediterranean diet, walking a few miles each day with the poodle, and I sleep like a teenager each night with vivid dreams. Great sleep is healing. Could it be my cure? With fingers crossed, I pray for a miracle.

chapter 43

TruDOSE™ Redux

If the human brain were so simple that we could understand it, we would be so simple that we couldn't.
—Emerson W. Pugh[72]

There is a thirty-year experience of using platelet rich plasma for wound healing, intra-articular joint injections for sports injuries and osteoarthritis, and subcutaneous injections into the scalp for hair growth. TruDOSE is a patented treatment of PRP (Platelet Rich Plasma), with a specific dose of the patient's own platelets introduced IVP (intravenous push), to treat the body systemically. How does the body prioritize where healing is required? There is a somatic hierarchy based on the relative importance of vital organs—brain, heart, and lungs. I am glad to know that my storm-ravaged brain is first in line for rejuvenation. Joints and skin are less important targets for platelets since problems upstream are vital for patient survival. If skin was the number one priority, we could all look marvelous in our coffins. I personally prefer to feel well while sporting a few wrinkles.

Why platelets? My first thought is that platelets form clots to prevent loss of blood from a breach of the skin. Yes, they do that. But they do not cause clotting unless it is necessary, or if there is an underlying clotting disorder. Platelets manage the relationship of blood components: hormones, cells, and neurotransmitters. The super-charged platelet rich plasma infusion helps the body reboot and rebalance blood components, so that healing occurs. PRP optimizes the innate ability of the body to heal. Responding to the human disease state, platelets carry 95 percent of the body's serotonin as well as 99 percent of Brain-Derived-Neurotrophic-Factor (BDNF), which is necessary for nerve regeneration.

PRP injections were initially used by sports medicine physicians to decrease healing time for professional athletes. PRP is a natural progression from the use of stem cells which are more difficult and painful to retrieve, yet with similar actions and results at a much lower cost. In 2002, it was said that stem cells would transform medicine. For certain cancers, this is true. And now, will PRP become the newest life-changing treatment? PRP recruits the body's own stem cells. No donors necessary. Using a patient's own body fluids to jump-start the healing process is worth a try. In 2015, Tapley Holland, a stem cell field expert embarked on a mission trip that opened a new avenue for healing. A young patient with a paralyzing spinal cord injury was treated with stem cells and PRP seven days post-accident. He recovered completely. A second young patient, twenty-one days post-spinal cord injury, was also treated with stem cells and PRP. Despite an outbreak of pseudomonas aeruginosa, (a gram-negative bacterium which can be lethal in patients with a weakened immune system), in the ICU, he survived and was able to walk again. Tapley said that the antimicrobial properties of PRP saved this patient while others in the ICU succumbed to the deadly bacterium. After this eye-opening experience, Tapley built software which became the foundation of TruDOSE, a means of properly dosing each patient based on their platelet count/ml and using AI to establish guidelines for individual medical conditions, through data derived from previously treated patients.

Sports stars such as golfer Tiger Woods and tennis great Raphael Nadal have had speedy recoveries from injuries with PRP treatments. Patients with severe alopecia have regrown hair, and a certain group of wealthy beauty mavens have used PRP in "vampire facials" for a more youthful appearance. But who and what will be treated with TruDOSE? So far, patients with Autism, Cerebral Palsy, Lyme Disease, Parkinson's Disease, Rheumatoid Arthritis. Why not chronic migraine?

While reading an article in *The Journal of Headache and Pain*, "Migraine and neuroinflammation: the inflammasome perspective," *(2021)* by Oguzhan Kursun, Muge Yemisci, Arn M.J.M. van den Maagdenberg, and Hulya Karatas,[73] I zero in on this new-to-me term—inflammasome. This is a large protein complex which plays a role in sensing inflammatory signals and triggers an innate immune response.

My brain is aflame and needs dousing to eliminate its pain. Why not tap into the healing potential of my body's own platelets? Since platelets travel throughout the bloodstream looking for things to repair, how about giving them a boost with a higher concentration? I like this strategy and there are no or minimal side effects.

One of my friends recently tried intra-articular PRP for her arthritic knee. She was disappointed that the $500 she spent did not produce a reduction in pain. I research online and find a Stanford trained sports medicine physician who explains everything a patient should know about PRP injections. Jeffrey Peng, M.D. says in his YouTube videos,[74] that "there is a critical number of cells necessary to incite healing." The concentration should be personalized to the patient. Currently, many physicians administering PRP into damaged knee joints are giving each patient the same volume, though the concentration of platelets is unknown. It may work for some, but what about that patient's physiology? How many platelets are present in each millimeter of a patient's blood? Dr. Peng says that "correct dosage is ten billion platelets with a 60ml blood draw." He recommends that a therapeutic PRP dose "is four to six times the baseline platelets for best results. Double spin in the centrifuge is necessary," he says. And for joint injections, imaging with ultrasound is imperative to hit target sites.

Does the patient have any underlying conditions which may interfere with platelet activity? If a patient takes NSAIDs (non-steroidal anti-inflammatories) prior to or in the weeks following PRP injection, these medications will inhibit platelet function, since they are anti-inflammatory, and inflammation is part of the healing process. Steroids interfere similarly. These drugs should be stopped one week before and six weeks following PRP to prevent interference with the liquid gold PRP. Metabolic health issues such as uncontrolled hypertension, diabetes, hypercholesterolemia, and obesity can also impair healing by their inflammatory states. Alcohol, tobacco, and cannabinoids should be avoided before and after treatment.

Nine and a half weeks out from my initial TruDOSE treatment, I travel across the state of Michigan for another. The neurosurgeon in this office reserves a few days each month to treat patients with TruDOSE. I make an appointment with a $600 deposit and show up early for my cure. A receptionist offers me a snack of fruit, cheese, and crackers. I wait about ninety minutes to be seen and the neurosurgeon visits while I wait for preparation of my personalized dose of PRP. He pokes me in the lower back since I have noted spinal stenosis on my intake form as well as chronic migraine. He is satisfied that my sacroiliac joint is not yet a candidate for surgery since I do not leap off the exam table during his probing. He mentions ozone therapy (which I Google on the spot) without receiving any reassurance that it may be worth trying to regain a pain-free golf swing. During the long wait, I drink several bottles of water. It is a hot day, and I have been reminded a few times to hydrate before the procedure. On one of my trips to the loo, I dislodge the catheter in my right arm. When the technician returns with the large syringe of my liquid gold, she first attempts to flush the line with saline, and I nearly jump off the table. "It is no longer in my vein," I say. She withdraws the misplaced catheter, and I suggest using the left arm for the IV push. After this mishap I become dizzy and spend another half hour recovering, with my right arm swollen and throbbing.

I left home this morning at 9:30 am for the appointment and finally pull into my driveway at 7:30 pm. After 265 miles of driving around road construction in Grand Rapids, Lansing, and Flint, I feel lousy, my right arm is killing me, and I have a whopper migraine. Otherwise, life is fine-oh-fine. Maybe a driver should be hired for a subsequent treatment.

The Data: In the past four weeks since the second TruDOSE therapy, I have endured *eleven days with migraine*. However, I have also experienced what is called a Herxheimer reaction, feeling achy and fluish for several days. After my first treatment, I did not experience this type of reaction though I am told that this is a common response. But since I felt a lot better after the first dose, maybe I should head back to Louisville in sixty days for a repeat treatment of Blue Grass magic.

TruDOSE in Grand Blanc costs $1,450 plus $10 per month to join the non-optional The Body Healthcare group. This reminds me of joining a "club" at Deer Valley ski area in Utah to enjoy an après ski libation in a dry county. Interesting concept. After a few months of automatic withdrawals from my checking account, I cancel this unnecessary subscription.

So how is it working for me? A more honest accounting is this: January 2024, *twenty-one migraine days* on very expensive Qulipta as a preventative; February, *eighteen migraine days*, while still on Qulipta; March, *eleven migraine days* without Qulipta and my first TruDOSE administered on March 16; April, *nine migraine days*; May, *ten migraine days* with a second TruDOSE on May 21; June, *eleven migraine days*; July, *eight migraine days*; August, *eight migraine days* and my sleep is still improving. The trend is slightly encouraging.

chapter 44

MAY THE THIRD TIME BE MY CHARM

The human brain has 100 billion neurons, each neuron connected to 10 thousand other neurons. Sitting on your shoulders is the most complicated object in the known universe.
—Michio Kaku[75]

Why am I surprised that my brain is the source of my pain, and the keeper of all my joy? Joy hides in every cell and bursts forth like a sunflower seeking the sun when I am without pain. As clouds part, my brainstorm lifts, and once again I tap into the consciousness I share with this world, transcending past pain and sorrow.

After breakfast on September 12, 2024, I ingest frovatriptan at 8 am for a migraine in progress and slap together a PBJ on homemade rosemary rye bread. This is insurance food, to be consumed in the car in case I do not have time for a real lunch. Low blood sugar is a migraine trigger. I hydrate with water and electrolytes, and dose myself with a second coffee as I travel across the state to the Bio Energy Medical Center. The traffic sucks. It is even worse than the last time. Construction sites, with no work crews present, shut down lanes of I-96 traffic near Grand Rapids, Lansing, and I-94 into Ann Arbor. Captive motorists inch along on the road's corduroy shoulder and my travel time is increased by an extra sixty minutes or more each way. Big Gretch, (Michigan's governor Gretchen Whitmer) vowed to "fix the damn roads" six years ago as her gubernatorial campaign pledge. *Let's rip 'em up and leave 'em until I can force a juicy gas tax increase to pay for it.* She did not say this part out loud, but it is repeated by motorists across the state while they sit seething in traffic. I sigh and eye my humble sandwich. I had been looking forward to tastier fare at a twee tea shop in Ann Arbor, but my hourglass is draining faster than the flow of traffic. I am crabby and impatient as I consider the upcoming TruDOSE treatment at a new-to-me clinic.

The Bio Energy Clinic is in an industrial park near the expressway. No frills, but the intake nurse practitioner spends an hour going over my medical history after reviewing my online details. And this caring nurse calls me on two subsequent weeks to monitor my symptoms after treatment. I am sure that the office bills Medicare for these calls, but it feels more holistic. I feel cared for as a person, not just a source of income.

The last clinic was not so concerned about my total health. The neurosurgery office where I received my second TruDOSE treatment called once. Since I was unable to take the call, I left two messages for the PA but never received a call back. The blown IV, an odd offer of ozone injections for my spinal stenosis, and the $10 monthly bill to my credit card for nothing tangible led me away from this site. The first clinic in Kentucky was fine; the nurse called me a couple of weeks post treatment to check on me, but the six-hour drive is not ideal.

The actual treatment at the Bio Energy Clinic is easy and relatively quick. One hour in a recliner for prep, centrifuging, and administration of my PRP. Instead of a finger-stick to withdraw initial blood for assessing my current platelet concentration, Karen expertly inserts an IV catheter into the antecubital vein, withdraws a few mls of blood, and runs it through the Tru-DOSE computer. She returns in a few minutes after receiving AI-generated information, which prescribes the volume of blood necessary for a proper dose of platelets. My first two treatments involved larger blood draws, but perhaps the finger stick is not an accurate way to measure my platelet concentration. Since I have Raynaud's, it is difficult to squeeze enough blood from my cold fingers. It took several minutes of milking the lanced digit to obtain a sufficient volume of blood for a test. I believe that the sample obtained was not entirely blood; it was likely diluted by extracellular fluid, resulting in an erroneous platelet count. Hence, a larger volume of blood may have been calculated (via the finger-stick method) as necessary to obtain the proper dose of platelets. I believe that the first clinic withdrew four x 60ml of blood, the second clinic withdrew Four x 60ml of blood, and the third clinic withdrew two x 50ml of blood, all purporting to give me the correct dose of PRP. I believe that testing by finger stick is not accurate, and it is also uncomfortable for the patient. With one poke to place the catheter, a more accurate platelet concentration is obtained from blood withdrawn directly from the vein. Little things make a big difference.

This treatment was a few weeks ago, and once again I feel slammed by a Herxheimer reaction, feeling achy and exhausted, like I am fighting something. I am. Let's hope this battle is focused on diminishing the brainstorm. September, *seven migraine days*. October, *five migraine days*. The weather has been unusually dry, with minor barometric pressure fluctuations, and my fingers are crossed. It is early in this experiment: three treatments with my own super-charged platelets in March, June, and September. I will reserve judgement until twelve months have passed. Overturning decades of my brain defaulting to brainstorm may take time. I am working on patience and know that I have nothing to lose but pain as I use everything I can to overcome chronic migraine. There are glimmers of hope where the light gets in.

chapter 45

The Verdict

Men ought to know that from the brain, and from the brain only, arise our pleasures, joys, laughter, and jests, as well as sorrows, pains, griefs, and tears.
—Hippocrates[76]

While driving home after taking care of her 92-year-old mother (my mother's sister), who shows symptoms of dementia, my cousin Karen experienced a sudden loss of vision and a severe headache. At age 65, this was her first migraine episode, most likely induced by an overload of stress. She says that two of her sisters have experienced occasional auras lasting for twenty-thirty minutes, with loss of half of their vision in one eye, but without head pain. Karen's presentation is bilateral and near blindness. She says that in the emergency room, she saw the attending physician with two blurry heads. It appears that a familial tendency toward migraine, along with too much stress, nudged my dear cousin into this scary circumstance. It has been about five weeks since her initial migraine manifestation, and her pain has diminished from ten to two on a scale of 1-10, but her vision is still abnormal. She is unable to work or drive safely. I suggest a headache specialty clinic within an hour of her home. They may start her on a steroid taper to break up the daily headache, though further investigation is warranted.

Several months later I hear that Karen is about to undergo a second knee replacement procedure. I call her and tell her I will pray for a great result and a full recovery. And then I ask about her migraine. She says, "It vanished. I've been healed." As a cradle Catholic, I believe in the power of prayer though I have reserved my prayers for others. Perhaps it is time that I begin to pray for my own healing.

Every migraineur has her own story and treatment must be individualized. But universally, migraineurs should be vigilant in avoiding triggers, learn coping mechanisms for stressors, ensure adequate hydration, rest, ice the painful area, take appropriate supplements such as magnesium, and exercise caution to prevent MOH (medication overuse headache) from daily use of acetaminophen, NSAIDs, triptans, etc.

There is not yet a cure for migraine. We are inching closer, but I do not think it will happen during my lifetime. A cure may be found in a gene-splicing procedure, an immunotherapy intervention, or a brain transplant engineered by a 3-D printer. Just kidding about the last item, though I may get in touch with Elon Musk and present the case for a study using his Neuralink™ brain implant for chronic migraine. For so many, a migraine cure would be light-years better than a trip to Mars. And I read a March 2024 article in *Scientific American* titled "Most Astronauts Get Space Headaches. Scientists Want to Know Why" by Joanna Thompson. The author says, "Headaches are a common and recurring problem in space, even for astronauts that don't experience them on earth." [77] Musk says he likes to take the fiction out of science fiction. *Et tu,* Elon. This could be your next gift to the world: a cure for brainstorm, on earth as well as in space. Still, I am heartened by the improved treatments available today when I look back on my first encounter with migraine in the 1960s and a near-overdose of aspirin, without any relief.

    Botox, as a nerve-numbing preventative, with a triptan (currently frovatriptan), plus a gram of acetaminophen, are my go-to storm chasers. They are not perfect, somewhat effective, but they beat the pants off opioids, trepanning, and bloodletting. Though medicine has come a long way, we have a few more miles to go. It is tough to endure this malady. It is more than *just a headache*, and it deserves intensive and continuing research. I believe we are approaching a satisfying brainstorm reboot. Let's stay in touch as we seek our cure. It is a great time to be alive as science directs glimmers of light into our black box brains.

    Wishing you peaceful nights and pain-free days.

Learn to *Lean*

Like trees we learn to *lean* with the breeze,
    Preparing for autumn winds and January gales.
Anchoring roots allow us to *sway* ~
    though if we turn brittle, we b-r-e-a-k.

Leaden limbs crash to earth,
    decompose into forest floor,
        as woodpeckers tattoo our skins.

In winter our sap slows its flow~
    While we sleep beneath blankets
        of lichen, sere leaves, and sometimes snow.

Reborn in spring as saplings,
    arisen from the forest floor,
        we greet each fresh breeze,
            and learn to *lean* and *sway* again.

—Susan P. Ryan

You'll miss 100% of the shots that you never take.
—Wayne Gretzky[78]

Do not accept defeat.
—Bruce Lee.[79]

Postscript

It has been twelve months since my first TruDOSE PRP treatment on March 16, 2024. Six weeks later I received another dose of my very own golden colored super-charged platelet-rich serum on May 21 and on September 12 my third dose. I have taken the winter off since I have been feeling better than usual. My migraine days are as follows: September 7 days, October 5 days, November 9 days, December 6 days, January 4 days, February 4 days, March 5 days. I cannot call this a cure yet, but I like the trend so far and there are longer gaps between my migraine days. Though I was hoping for total remission in a year, I realize that it took decades for my migraines to reach the chronic level. Any cure, a retraining and remodeling of my brain may take a few more treatments. Today, I made a $600 deposit for my next TruDOSE appointment scheduled for April 1. I will keep you posted.

"It is part of the cure to wish to be cured."
—Seneca

Glossary of Terms

acute migraine: episodic migraine occurring on less than fifteen days per month.

ADD: Attention Deficit Disorder, also called ADHD, Attention Deficit Hyperactivity Disorder. A medically diagnosed chronic condition; includes difficulty in maintaining attention, controlling hyperactivity, and impulsiveness.

adsorb: particles from one substance adhere onto the surface of another.

anticholinergic: substances that block acetylcholine, a neurotransmitter.

aphasia: loss or impairment in spoken language.

atrial fibrillation (AF): rapid and irregular beating of the upper chambers of the heart. Symptoms include fainting, dizziness, chest pain, shortness of breath. Can be caused by high blood pressure, valvular heat disease, obesity, smoking, sleep apnea, or aging. AF patients may take anticoagulants and/or antiplatelet drugs to prevent stroke.

aura: migraine aura refers to a sensory, motor, or visual disturbance; considered to be the second stage of migraine.

black box warning: Based on clinical data or serious animal toxicity, a black box warning means that an adverse reaction may lead to death or serious injury. It is the FDA's most serious warning for drugs and medical devices.

BDNF: brain derived neurotrophic factor; a protein in the growth factor family. Essential for cell survival, mood related behaviors, synaptic (nerve ending) plasticity, and involved in the control of eating and drinking. Can be affected by diet: high fat or high sugar consumption can interfere with normal functioning of BDNF.

BMI: Body Mass Index is a means of measuring body fat in adults based on weight and height. There are on-line calculators or the formula for self-calculation is: BMI=weight in pounds divided by height in inches, squared, and multiplied by 703 as the conversion factor when using pounds and inches.

CAT scan: computed axial tomography; also called CT scan. Uses high dose x-ray (ionizing radiation) to create images of the body for diagnosis.

Cefaly: FDA-approved medical device for treatment of migraine. It is an external TENS (trans-cutaneous electrical nerve stimulation) unit, which specifically acts on the trigeminal nerve.

CBD: cannabidiol, one of one-hundred-thirteen identified cannabinoids in the cannabis plant. Popular as a *possible* treatment for anxiety, depression, insomnia, pain, and PTSD.

Glossary of Terms

charcoal tablets: as charcoal moves through the gastrointestinal tract it adsorbs harmful substances.

CGRP Inhibitor: a class of drugs known as calcitonin-gene-related-peptide inhibitors; used as migraine preventatives.

chi: also **qi;** vital life force in traditional Chinese medicine, thought to flow throughout the body along specific meridians.

chronic migraine: episodic migraine is converted to chronic when a patient experiences migraine on fifteen or more days in a month for at least three months.

cluster headache: rare condition of one-sided, severe headaches. They usually follow a pattern of a particular time of day. They can linger for months, disappear for long stretches, then reappear.

colic: refers to infantile condition of digestive pain, manifested by unconsolable crying.

CoQ10: coenzyme Q-10, found in most cells of the human body; vital for metabolism; antioxidant, biochemical co-factor, energy-producer. Medical uses: as a supplement for heart health, in reducing blood pressure and improving symptoms of congestive heart failure; helps reduce cholesterol levels in patients with diabetes; may reduce frequency of migraines.

cortical spreading depression: in migraine, this refers to a depolarization wave through the cerebral cortex, underlying the aura phase.

CRP: C-Reactive Protein blood test measures inflammation in the human body.

cyberchondria: unfounded concern regarding symptoms, due to a review of literature on-line.

DC: order to discontinue a treatment

FODMAPs: fermentable oligosaccharides, disaccharides, monosaccharides, and polyols; a group of carbohydrates that are not well absorbed in the gut. FODMAPS may cause digestive issues in some patients as they ferment in the large intestine, expanding and causing discomfort.

GLP-1: Glucagon-like-peptide-1 is produced in the intestine. It can decrease blood sugar levels by enhancing secretion of insulin. A class of GLP-1 drugs has been developed to mimic this activity and has resulted in better control of type two diabetes, weight loss, and many other positive side effects.

H & P: History and Physical exam, conducted by medical staff in assessing a patient.

HEPA: High Efficiency Particulate Air (filter), refers to an air filter that can trap very small harmful particles such as pet dander, dust, mold, pollen, and other allergens. Designed to capture 99.7 percent of all particles 0.3 microns or smaller; this will help a consumer breathe easier and sleep better.

Herxheimer Reaction: aka Jarisch-Herxheimer (JHR) or "herxing." An elevated immune response with symptoms of chills, fever, headache, skin rash. Caused by a die-off of an infective organism.

homeopathy: an alternative medicine that employs highly diluted substances to stimulate the body to heal.

HBOT: hyperbaric oxygen treatment. A patient breathes pure oxygen at elevated pressure in an enclosed chamber for several conditions: to speed up healing of wounds, gangrene, carbon monoxide poisoning, or "the bends," experienced by deep sea divers suffering from rapid pressure change.

HRT: hormone replacement therapy.

hyperemesis: severe nausea and vomiting which can occur during pregnancy or as a result of cannabis use. Patients may become dehydrated and require IV fluids.

IBS: irritable bowel syndrome. Not curable per se, but symptoms can be managed by avoiding FODMAPs and other foods which may trigger symptoms of diarrhea, bloating, constipation.

IM: intramuscular route of administration.

inflammasome: a multi-protein danger sensing complex, which instigates the body's inflammatory response. It can be instrumental in healing, or when overactive, can lead to a range of diseases such as MS and Alzheimer's.

indica: a cannabis strain, from a shorter plant, considered to be relaxing versus sativa's energizing effects.

IVP: intravenous push, a method of giving a bolus of undiluted medication directly into the blood stream.

kelpie: from Scottish folklore; a shape-shifting water spirit that can appear as a grey or white horse with a dripping mane; or a human luring people to their death.

ketogenesis: chemical process that produces ketones when there are insufficient carbohydrates available for energy production.

Krebs Cycle: aka the citric acid cycle; a series of biochemical reactions which release energy stored in nutrients.

lacrimal duct: tear duct.

leaky gut syndrome: considered a hypothetical condition by mainstream medicine in which intestines become permeable to toxins that leak into the bloodstream. Treatment includes avoidance of inflammation by elimination from the diet of processed foods, alcohol, allergens, or foods which evoke sensitivities. Leaky gut has been suspected as a cause of autoimmune diseases, but we await clinical studies.

L-Glutamine: the most abundant amino acid in the human body. Used as a supplement to strengthen the gut lining. Should be avoided in patients with psychiatric disorders or a history of seizures; also, should be avoided in patients with decreased kidney function.

MAOI: Monoamine oxidase inhibitor; class of antidepressant drugs which change brain chemistry. Considered a class of antidepressants to be used only when other drugs have failed. Patients on these drugs should avoid tyramine-laden foods, since MAOIs prevent the breakdown of tyramine in the body, causing dangerously high blood pressure.

MOH: medication overuse headache, also known as "rebound headache." This is considered a secondary headache caused by ingesting an acute treatment too often. The neurons become acclimated to this treatment and rebel when it is withheld. It is recommended to restrict pain medications, whether prescription or over the counter, and also triptans, to two-three days per week and ten days maximum per month. Otherwise MOH may ensue, and an acute migraine patient is on her way to becoming "chronic."

moiety: in pharmacology, the part of the molecule responsible for the activity of the drug.

MRI: magnetic resonance imaging. Uses radio waves and a very strong magnetic field to produce sharp images inside the body. No radiation involved. Non-invasive except for the noise. I recommend using headphones offered by the MRI technician and requesting soothing jazz as a distraction. Claustrophobics should keep their eyes closed.

MSG: monosodium glutamate. A naturally occuring (in certain foods) chemical used as a flavor enhancer that the Food and Drug Administration has "recognized as safe." Despite its delicious umami taste, a sensitive migraineur may find MSG to be a trigger. It is considered a neurotoxin which enters the brain through the mouth and throat and may overstimulate a migraineur's already fatigued neurons. It may be listed as "natural flavoring" on processed food labels.

naturopathic: according to the American Association of Naturopathic Physicians: "Naturopathic Physicians are educated and trained in accredited naturopathic medical colleges." They are interested in optimizing health by "supporting the person's inherent self-healing process." By identifying "underlying causes of illness, [they] develop personalized plans to address them."

neuroplasticity: The ability of the brain to remodel itself in response to learning, experience, or following an injury.

niacin: Vitamin B-3, a water-soluble vitamin that converts food into energy. Occurs naturally and is available as a dietary supplement.

NSAID: Nonsteroidal Anti-Inflammatory Drug. Non-opioid analgesic for mild to moderate pain, also reduces inflammation, fever. Examples are naproxen, ibuprofen, and aspirin.

NPO: medical abbreviation for *nil per os*, meaning nothing by mouth.

OC: oral contraceptive.

Osteoporosis: medical condition of brittle bones, caused by hormonal change, deficiency of Vitamin D, or excessive steroid use.

OTC: over the counter; products available without a prescription, such as aspirin and many nutritional supplements and vitamins.

pathophysiology: study of abnormalities in bodily functions, looking for causes and consequences of a particular disease process.

pericardial tamponade: occurs when fluid in the pericardial sac collects and compresses the heart.

PFO: Patent Foramen Ovale. An opening in the septum between the atria (upper right and left sides) of the heart. PFO is normal in utero, to allow blood to bypass the fetal lungs, which do not work until air is inhaled at birth. The PFO usually closes after birth, though in about twenty-five percent of the population, it may remain. If small, it may be undetected and inconsequential.

phenotype: physical characteristics of an individual resulting from the environmental effects acting on genotype.

phonophobia: sensitivity to sound.

photophobia: sensitivity to light.

PICC Line: Peripherally Inserted Central Catheter. A long flexible tube that is inserted into a vein usually in the arm for administration of fluids and drugs.

polypharmacy: using five or more prescription drugs. It may lead to serious adverse reactions.

PRP: Platelet Rich Plasma. Patients are treated with their own platelets for healing and tissue regeneration. The patient's blood is withdrawn and spun in a centrifuge, separating the platelets from other blood components. The platelet-rich top layer is returned to the patient, enhancing healing and tissue regeneration.

PRN: pro re nata, Latin abbreviation for "as the thing is needed." PRN meds are taken only as needed, not on a regular schedule.

prodrome: an early symptom. In migraine, the first phase of migraine which can last a day or two before the head pain.

Red Haven peaches: introduced by Stanley Johnson in South Haven, Michigan in 1940. Freestone, juicy, rich in flavor, and nearly fuzz-less. As a former resident of South Haven and a peach connoisseur, I consider them to be perfectly peachy.

RLS: restless legs syndrome: a neurological disorder causing an urge to move the legs, often interfering with sleep. Triggers include consumption of alcohol, caffeine, nicotine, some medications, stress. Treatment includes Vitamin D and/or iron supplementation (check levels prior), antiseizure drugs, dopamine agonists, regular exercise, but not close to bedtime.

sativa: tall, thin cannabis plant. The drug action of sativa is more invigorating and energizing than indica.

serotonin syndrome: a serious drug reaction which can occur when certain drugs such as some antidepressants interact with other drugs including over the counter supplements and cause a build-up of serotonin. Too much serotonin (a neurotransmitter) can cause mild symptoms like diarrhea and nausea, while severe symptoms like elevated blood pressure, rapid heart rate, fever, and seizure can be fatal if not recognized and treated.

shinrin-yoku: Japanese therapeutic practice of forest bathing; connecting with nature for relaxation.

SJS: Stevens-Johnson Syndrome: a rare, very serious reaction to a medication or infection, causing a medical crisis. It may start as a rash and progress to multi-organ failure.

sphenopalatine ganglion block: SPG; administration of a local anesthetic through a catheter to the sphenopalatine ganglion, the nerves behind the nasal passages, which are connected to the trigeminal nerves and involved in migraine pain.

sphyganomometer: a device to measure blood pressure by means of an inflatable cuff which collapses and releases an artery in a controlled way.

SSRI: selective serotonin reuptake inhibitor. A class of drugs mainly used as antidepressants. The drug works by inhibiting the reabsorption of serotonin by neurons, allowing a buildup of this neurotransmitter.

sternocleidomastoid: the largest muscle on the front of the neck.

Tapley Holland: developer of TruDOSE PRP therapy.

TCA: tricyclic antidepressant. An older class of antidepressants developed in the 1950s. Still available and used also for chronic pain, migraine, insomnia, fibromyalgia, OCD, anxiety.

TENS unit: transcutaneous electrical nerve stimulator. A small battery-operated device which uses a mild electrical current to block pain transmission, stimulate healing after injury or surgery, and reduce inflammation.

THC: Tetrahydrocannabinol; chemical cause of most of the psychological effects of cannabis.

TMJ: temporomandibular joint. Joint in front of each ear which connects the mandible (lower jaw) to the skull.

trigeminal nerves: a pair of large cranial nerves (#5) that innervate either side of the face.

trigger point injections: a therapeutic method to release muscle knots (myofascial trigger points) with either dry needling or injection of lidocaine (anesthetic).

triptan: a class of tryptamine-based drugs (5HT-1) used as abortive medication in migraine and cluster headache. Triptans should not be used by patients taking SSRI drugs to avoid serotonin syndrome.

TruDOSE®: IV platelet rich plasma therapy which calibrates the dosage of a patient's own platelets to boost the immune system so that the body can heal itself.

Type A: personality that is organized, goal-oriented, competitive, driven to succeed. Not one to waste time, nor laid-back; may be a perfectionist. Can lead to health issues of headache persistence, insomnia, digestive problems.

venipuncturist: medical technician trained in entering a patient's vein to withdraw blood or administer an IV.

Bibliography

Brink, Martin. *The Migraine Revolution: Scientific Guide to Effective Treatment and Permanent Headache Relief.* Robina, Queensland, Australia: Body, Mind, and Brain, 2012.

Bucholz, David. *Heal Your Headache: The 1,2,3 Program for taking charge of your pain.* New York: Workman Publishing, 2002.

Cohen, Jay. *The Magnesium Solution for Migraine Headaches: How to use Magnesium to Prevent and Relieve Migraine and Cluster Headaches Naturally.* Garden City Park, NY: Square One Publishers, 2004.

Cowan, Robert. *The Keeler Migraine Method: A Groundbreaking, Individualized Treatment Program from the Renowned Headache Clinic.* New York: Avery, 2008.

D'Adamo, Peter, J. with Whitney, Catherine. *Eat Right 4 Your Type: The Individualized Blood Type Diet Solution: 4 Blood Types, 4 diets.* New York: Penguin, 1996.

DeLaune, Valerie. *Trigger Point Therapy for Headaches and Migraines: Your Self-Treatment Workbook for Pain Relief.* Oakland, CA: New Harbinger Publications, 2008.

Diamond, Seymour and Franklin, Mary. *Headache Through the Ages.* West Islip, NY: Professional Communications, 2005.

Dzugan, Sergey and Mitchell, Deborah. *The Migraine Cure: How to Banish the Curse of Migraines Using a Totally Effective, Safe, Clinically Proven Yet Drug-Free Medical Breakthrough.* St Paul, MN: Dragon Door Publications, 2006.

Eban, Katherine. *Bottle of Lies: The Inside Story of the Generic Drug Boom.* New York: HarperCollins Publishers, 2019.

Ellison, Amanda. *Splitting: The Inside Story on Headaches.* London: Green Tree, Bloomsbury Publishing Plc., 2020.

Fancher, Danielle Newport. *10: A Memoir of Migraine Survival.* Self-Published, 2018.

Fox, Dennis and Rejaunier, Jeanne. *The Complete Idiot's Guide to Migraines and Other Headaches.* Indianapolis, IN: Alpha Books, 2000.

Ivker, Robert, S. and Nelson, Todd. *Headache Survival: The Holistic Medical Treatment Program for Migraine, Tension, and Cluster Headaches.* New York: Putnam, 2002.

Jones, Andrew. *The Natural Cure to your Migraine Headache: What the Big Companies Don't Want You to Know.* Self-Published, 2009.

Kamen, Paula. *All In My Head: An Epic Quest to Cure an Unrelenting, Totally Unreasonable, and Only Slightly Enlightening Headache.* Cambridge, MA: Da Capo Press, 2005.

Leroux, Elizabeth. *Migraines: More Than a Headache.* Toronto, Ontario, Canada: Dundurn, 2016.

Levy, Andrew. *A Brain Wider Than the Sky: A Migraine Diary.* New York: Simon and Schuster, 2009.

Martelletti, Paolo, Editor. *Migraine in Medicine: A Machine-Generated Overview of Current Research.* Cham, Switzerland: Springer, 2022.

Mauskop, Alexander. *The End of Migraines: 150 Ways to Stop Your Pain.* New York: Self-Published, 2022.

BIBLIOGRAPHY

Means, Casey. *Good Energy: The Surprising Connection Between Metabolism and Limitless Health.* New York: Avery, 2024.

Milne, Robert and More, Blake, with Goldberg, Burton. *Headaches: Headaches Can Be Eliminated Using Natural Therapies.* Tiburon, CA: Future Medicine Publishing, 1997.

Nasiuk, Dariusz J., *PRP—Platelet Rich Plasma: A New Paradigm of Regenerative Medicine.* Master Printing, 2023.

Reed, Abby J., *The Color of Pain: The Intersection of Migraine, Art, and Faith.* Monee, IL: Polaris Creations, 2022.

Sacks, Oliver. *Migraine.* New York: Vintage, 1999.

Sacks, Oliver. *The River of Consciousness.* New York: Alfred A. Knopf, 2017.

Shifflett, C.M. *Migraine Brains and Bodies: A Comprehensive Guide to Solving the Mystery of Your Migraines.* Sewickley, PA: Round Earth Publishing, 2011.

Slater, Lauren. *Blue Dreams: The Science and the Story of the Drugs That Changed Our Minds.* New York: Hachette Books, 2018.

Stanton, Angela. *Fighting the Migraine Epidemic: Complete Guide, How to Treat and Prevent Migraines Without Medicines.* North Charleston, SC: Create Space Independent Publishing Platform, 2017.

Walker, Matthew. *Why We Sleep: Unlocking the Power of Sleep.* New York: Scribner, 2017.

Warraich, Haider. *The Song of Our Scars: The Untold Story of Pain.* New York: Basic Books, 2022.

Wolf, Alicia. *The Dizzy Cook: Managing Migraine with More than 90 Comforting Recipes and Lifestyle Tips.* WestMarginPress.com, 2020.

Endnotes

1. "Many a trip continues long after movement in time and space has ceased." John Steinbeck, *Travels With Charley: In Search of America*. (1902-1968).
2. "Migraine and other headache disorders," World Health Organization, March 6, 2024; https://www.who.int/news-room/fact-sheets/detail/headache-disorders.
3. *Why We Sleep*. Matthew Walker, neuroscientist. (born 1974).
4. "I'm just glad to be feeling better. I really thought I'd be seeing Elvis soon." https://www.Flagging down the double E's.com/p/i-really-thought-id-be-seeing-elvis. Bob Dylan, American singer, songwriter, musician, author. (born 1941).
5. "Every day may not be good, but there is something good in every day." Alice Morse Earle, American writer and historian. (1851-1911).
6. "Those things that hurt instruct." Benjamin Franklin, Founding Father of the United States, writer, scientist, inventor, diplomat, publisher, philosopher. (1706-1790).
7. Chronic migraine risk factors. International Headache Society, London based organization founded in 1981.
8. "Biology gives you a brain. Life turns it into a mind." Jeffrey Eugenides, *Middlesex*. American novelist and short story writer. (born 1960).
9. "Never look back unless you are planning to go that way." Henry David Thoreau, American naturalist, philosopher, poet, essayist. (1817-1862).
10. "The natural healing force within each of us is the greatest force in getting well." Hippocrates, the "Father of Medicine," ancient Greek physician and philosopher. (circa 460-370BC).
11. "Be not simply good. Be good for something." Mahatma Gandhi, Indian lawyer, anti-colonial nationalist and political ethicist who espoused non-violent resistance in the successful campaign for India's independence from Britain. (1869-1948).
12. "The trouble with retirement is that you never get a day off." Abe Lemons, American college basketball coach. (1922-2002).

13 "A happy life consists not in the absence, but in the mastery of hardships." Helen Keller, American author and disability rights activist. (1880-1968).
14 "Do you love life? Then do not squander time, for that is the stuff life is made of." Benjamin Franklin. Ibid.
15 "Fear not death, for the sooner we die the longer we will be immortal." Benjamin Franklin, Ibid.
16 "Poison is in everything, and no thing is without poison. The dosage makes it either a poison or a remedy." Paracelsus, "The Father of Toxicology." Swiss physician, alchemist, lay theologian, philosopher. (1493-1551).
17 "I saw the angel and carved until I set him free." Michelangelo, Italian sculptor, painter, architect, and poet. (1475-1564).
18 "When many remedies are proposed for a disease, it means that the disease is incurable." Anton Chekhov, *The Cherry Orchard*," Act 1, (1904). Russian writer. (1860-1904).
19 *The Little Shop of Horrors*, film by Frank Oz and Howard Ashman,1986.
20 "Your brain has the power to modify pain perception." Wim Hof, Dutch author of "The Wim Hof Method: Activate Your Full Human Potential," motivational speaker
21 "Our greatest human adventure is the evolution of consciousness. We are in this world to enlarge the soul, liberate the spirit, and light up the brain." Tom Robbins, *Wild Ducks Flying Backward*. 2005. American author. (born 1932).
22 Mary Wollstonecraft Shelley, *Frankenstein*. First published in 1818. First science fiction novel. (1797-1851).
23 "All experience is great, providing you live through it. If it kills you, you've gone too far." Alice Neel. American visual artist, painter. (1900-1984).
24 "Suffering is the entrance to the person. It is the door to something larger." Rumi. Islamic scholar, poet, theologian. (1207-1273).
25 "Organic chemistry is the chemistry of carbon. Biochemistry is the study of carbon compounds that crawl." Mike Adams, aka "Health Ranger," founder of NaturalNews.com., author, inventor, publisher, podcaster.
26 "Glory lies in the attempt to reach one's goal and not in reaching it." Mahatma Gandhi, Ibid.
27 Petoskey stones from Lake Michigan show exquisite fossil formations when polished.
28 "The greater the dark, the easier to be a star." Stanislaw Jerzey Lec, Polish writer, Holocaust survivor. (1909-1966).
29 "If this is coffee, please bring me some tea; but if this is tea, please bring me some coffee." Abraham Lincoln, 16th American president. (1809-1865).
30 American Diabetes Association. *Diabetes Food Hub*. January 23, 2024."Six Tea-rrific Ways to Use Tea in Diabetes-Friendly Cooking), Jackie Newgent, RDN, CDN.
31 "Repression of calcitonin gene-related peptide expression in trigeminal neurons by a Theobroma cacao extract" by Marcie J. Abbey, Vinit V. Patil, Carrie V. Vause, and Paul L. Durham, The Journal of Ethnopharmacology, 2008.

Endnotes

32 Habitual Consumption of Caffeine." Yasgur, Batya Swift. Medscape. February 19, 2024.
33 "The Cure for anything is salt water: sweat, tears, or the sea." Karen Blixen, "The Deluge of Norderney." 1934. Danish author, (1885-1962).
34 "As sickness is the greatest misery, so the greatest misery of sickness is solitude." John Donne, Devotion V Meditation. English metaphysical poet, scholar, soldier, cleric in the Church of England. (1572-1631).
35 "I was looking for something a lot heavier, yet melodic at the same time. Something different from heavy metal, a different attitude." Kurt Cobain, American musician, songwriter, founding member of grunge band Nirvana. (1967-1994).
36 "And into the forest I go—to lose my mind and find my soul." John Muir, Scottish born, American naturalist, author, environmental philosopher, botanist, zoologist, advocate for wilderness preservation. 'Father of National Parks." (1838-1914).
37 "Forest Bathing: A Retreat Can Boost Your Immunity." Allison Aubrey, Morning Edition, National Public Radio 7/17/14.
38 "*The secret to mindful travel? A walk in the woods.*" Sunny Fitzgerald. Nationalgeographic.com. *18 Oct. 2019.*
39 "The chief function of the body is to carry the head around." Thomas A. Edison, American inventor in the field of electricity. (1838-1914).
40 "A gem cannot be polished without friction, nor a man perfected without trials." Seneca. Philosopher, statesman, orator. (4 B.C.E.-65 C.E.).
42 "Type A evolved with agrarian society." Peter J. D'Adamo, Catherine Whitney, *Eat Right for Your Type: The Individualized Diet Solution to Staying Healthy, Living Longer, and Achieving Your Ideal Weight.* Introduction xvii. 1996.
43 Low Tyramine Diet for Individuals with Headache or Migraine. (headaches.org)_The National Headache Foundation.
44 'Glucose tolerance is impaired during migraine." "*The metabolic face of migraine—from pathophysiology to treatment,*" Elena C. Gross, Marco Lisicki, ...Jean Schoenen. *Nature Reviews Neurology*,15, 627-643, (2019).
45 "The world breaks everyone and afterward many are stronger at the broken places. But those that will not break, it kills." Ernest Hemingway, *A Farewell to Arms.* Ch. 34. 1929.(1899-1961).
46 Cross, Rob and Dillon, Karen, *The Microstress Effect: How Little Things Pile Up and Create Big Problems and What to Do About It.* Brighton, MA: Harvard Business Review Press. 2023.
47 "Progress is impossible without change, and those who cannot change their minds, cannot change anything." George Bernard Shaw, Irish playwright. (1856-1950).
48 Martelletti, Paolo, Ed. *Migraine in Medicine: A Machine-Generated Overview of Current Research.*
49 Martelletti, Ibid., 218-219.
50 Martelletti, Ibid., 227.
51 Martelletti, Ibid., 233.

52   Martelletti, Ibid., 554.
53   Martelletti, Ibid., 534.
54   "Let food be thy medicine and medicine thy food." Hippocrates, Ibid.
55   "Don't sweat the petty things and don't pet the sweaty things." George Carlin, American stand-up comedian, social critic, actor, author. (1937-2008).
56   "Exact etiology of migraine, uncertain, none of the hitherto postulated mechanisms sufficiently explain the pathogenesis of migraine." *Journal of Neurology, Psychiatry, and Brain Research*, Volume 31, February 2019.
57   "Throw me to the wolves and I will return leading the pack." Seneca, Roman philosopher, statesman, orator, and leading intellectual in the mid first century. (c.4 B.C.E.-65 C.E.).
58   "It's not what happens to you, but how you react to it that matters." Epictetus, Greek Stoic philosopher. (55-135 C.E.)
59   "Insanity is doing the same thing over and over and expecting different results." Albert Einstein, German born theoretical physicist. Developed the theory of relativity. (1879-1955).
60   "Inspiration arrives as a packet of material to be delivered." John Updike, American novelist, poet, story writer, art and literary critic. (1932-2009).
61   "Broca's area, located in the left hemisphere, is associated with speech production articulation." UCSF Speech and Language Weill Institute of Neurosciences.
62   "I give you bitter pills in sugar coating. The pills are harmless; the poison is in the sugar." Stanislaw Jerzey Lec. Ibid.
63   Katherine Eban, investigative journalist, *Bottle of Lies: The Inside Story of the Generic Drug Boom*. 2019.
64   Rena M. Conti, Ernst R. Berndy, Neriman Beste Kaygisiz, Yashna Shivdasani, *We Still Don't Know Who Makes This Drug*." Health Affairs Forefront. 7 Feb, 2020.
65   "Lend yourself to others but give yourself to yourself." Michel de Montaigne, French Renaissance philosopher, essayist. (1533-1592).
66   "I don't so much fear death as I do wasting life." Oliver Sacks, MD, neurologist, author, fellow migraineur.
67   Eight Zen-Living Tips that can Change Your Life. https://123junk.com>blog137.
68   "Embrace the suck." Shared by a retired United States Marine. It is military slang for acceptance of unpleasant, unavoidable circumstances, deemed necessary for advancement.
69   OLLI (Oschner Lifelong Learning Institute) course.
70   "It is necessary to keep one's compass in one's eyes and not in the hand, for the hands execute, but the eye judges." Michelangelo. Ibid.
71   March Madness refers to NCAA (National College Athletic Association) basketball playoff season.
72   "If the human brain were so simple that we could understand it, we would be so simple that we couldn't." Emerson W. Pugh, American research engineer and scientist. (born 1929).

Endnotes

73 "Migraine and neuroinflammation: the inflammasome response." Oguzhan Kursun, Muge Yemisci, Arn MJM van den Maagdenberg, and Hulya Karatas. The Journal of Headache and Pain, 2021.
74 Jeffrey Peng, MD, non-operating orthopedist with a YouTube channel focusing on non-surgical treatments for sports injuries.
75 "The human brain has 100 billion neurons, each neuron connected to ten thousand other neurons. Sitting on your shoulders is the most complicated object in the known universe." Michio Kaku, American physicist. (Born 1947).
76 "Men ought to know that from the brain, and from the brain only, arise our pleasures, joys, laughter, and jests, as well as sorrows, pains, griefs, and tears." Hippocrates. Ibid.
77 "Most Astronauts Get Space Headaches and Scientists Want to Know Why." Joanna Thompson, Scientific American, March, 2024.
78 "You'll miss 100% of the shots that you never take." Wayne Gretzky, Canadian-born, with an unmatched twenty-year career playing in the National Hockey League (NHL). (Born 1961).
79 "Do not accept defeat." Bruce Lee. Hong-Kong-American actor, martial artist, filmmaker, philosopher. (1940-1973).

Acknowledgments

On this journey through *Brainstorm*, I have been blessed with many helpers, including my first readers, Patricia Eulitz and Betsy Snider. I value their views from outside the storm and their attention to detail.

A special thank you to Dr. David Sherer for reading and commenting on my manuscript. As an anesthesiologist with your special insight into pain management and your author's eye, I value your generosity.

Writerly wisdom from students and faculty at Spalding University's Master of Fine Arts in Writing Program echoed through my *Brainstorm* as I composed these pages.

Thank you to my family—Patricia, Mary Ellen, Kathleen, Jim, Tim, and Kevin. Even though we live hours apart, I know that you each have an ear that is near.

I appreciate the care and kindness of healthcare professionals who work to ease the storms.

Thank you to my wise editor and publisher, Maryann Karinch, who kept me focused on the path, and for believing that *Brainstorm* is a story worth sharing.

Thank you fellow migraineurs, who allowed me to pick through your personal storms. You taught me that each person suffers in her own way, with a unique approach to calming her tempest. We are separate yet not alone.

Author Bio

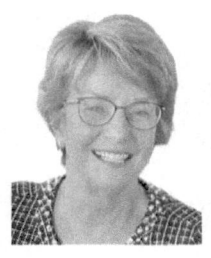

Susan P. Ryan is a graduate of the University of Michigan. She spent her career in the medical field, the last twenty-five years as a Heart Valve Specialist for Medtronic. After an early retirement, she received her MFA in Writing from Spalding University and decided to share her experience of enjoying a full life despite living with the number two cause of disability—chronic migraine. With optimism and humor, Susan shares what she has learned through oh-so-many trials, with the hope that it may lessen the load for others.

Susan lives in the Mitten State beside Lake Michigan with a sixty-two pound naughty companion, Vinny Van Poodle. Her essay "Proper Equipment" was awarded first prize for nonfiction sports writing and was published in winningwriters.com.

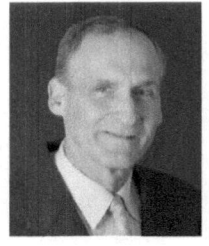Dr. David Sherer is an American physician, author, writer, blogger, medical-legal and patient safety expert. Through his work and the writing of his critically acclaimed book *Hospital Survival Guide*, he has helped people all over the world navigate the complexities of healthcare and lead healthier lives. His other recent books, *Hunger Hijack* and *What Your Doctor Isn't Telling You* further his mission of helping people understand how to take more control of their health and healthcare options. A retired anesthesiologist, Dave is a regular contributor to *Anesthesiology News*. His personal website is drdavidsherer.com.

www.ingramcontent.com/pod-product-compliance
Lightning Source LLC
Chambersburg PA
CBHW020048170426
43199CB00009B/210